Monographs in Human Genetics

Vol. 20

Series Editor

Michael Schmid Würzburg

Genetics of Deafness

Volume Editors

Barbara Vona Würzburg

Thomas Haaf Würzburg

14 figures, 4 in color, and 18 tables, 2016

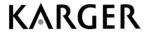

Basel · Freiburg · Paris · London · New York · Chennai · New Delhi ·
Bangkok · Beijing · Shanghai · Tokyo · Kuala Lumpur · Singapore · Sydney

Barbara Vona, PhD
Institute of Human Genetics
Biocentre
Julius-Maximilians-University
Am Hubland
DE–97074 Würzburg (Germany)

Thomas Haaf, MD
Institute of Human Genetics
Biocentre
Julius-Maximilians-University
Am Hubland
DE–97074 Würzburg (Germany)

Library of Congress Cataloging-in-Publication Data

Names: Vona, Barbara, editor. | Haaf, Thomas, editor.
Title: Genetics of deafness / volume editors, Barbara Vona, Thomas Haaf.
Other titles: Monographs in human genetics ; v. 20. 0077-0876
Description: Basel ; New York : Karger, 2016. | Series: Monographs in human
  genetics, ISSN 0077-0876 ; vol. 20 | Includes bibliographical references
  and indexes.
Identifiers: LCCN 2016009621| ISBN 9783318058550 (hard cover : alk. paper) |
  ISBN 9783318058567 (e-ISBN)
Subjects: | MESH: Hearing Loss--genetics
Classification: LCC RF291 | NLM WV 270 | DDC 617.8042--dc23 LC record available at
  http://lccn.loc.gov/2016009621

Bibliographic Indices. This publication is listed in bibliographic services, including Thomson Reuters indices.

© Copyright 2016 by S. Karger AG, P.O. Box, CH-4009 Basel (Switzerland)
www.karger.com
Printed in Germany on acid-free and non-aging paper (ISO 9706) by Kraft Druck, Ettlingen
ISSN 0077–0876
e-ISSN 1662–3835
ISBN 978–3–318–05855–0
e-ISBN 978–3–318–05856–7

Contents

Editorial

The objective of book series is to launch volumes on areas that are particularly interesting and in which there is a need for a thorough overview. Every time a new volume is published, the immediate task of editors responsible for a book series consists of finding and soliciting the assistance of one or more expert investigators to act as Guest Editors for the next volume. This is what I did when the last volume of *Monographs in Human Genetics* came off the press. And I did it for an unexpectedly long time, not coming to any reasonable result, but unaware of the fact that a solution was virtually present next door in our Department. During a fortuitous discussion on ongoing genetic services, I realized that a very important topic, the genetics of hearing loss, belongs to one of the main areas of interest of my colleagues Barbara Vona and Thomas Haaf. Both kindly accepted my invitation to act as Guest Editors and invited top researchers to contribute review articles. Barbara Vona took great pains in writing countless electronic messages to authors, coauthors and reviewers in order to keep this project going.

Thus, it is my great pleasure to introduce volume 20 of *Monographs in Human Genetics* devoted to 'Genetics of Deafness'. As with many other hereditary diseases, human genetics has achieved remarkable progress in the field of hearing loss, a condition with an extremely high world-wide prevalence. It should be reiterated here that the aim of *Monographs in Human Genetics* is to focus on important genetic diseases, their molecular causes and diagnosis, and their eventual prevention and clinical treatment. The present volume is a further example that meets this concept in a perfect way.

I express my deep gratitude to Barbara Vona and Thomas Haaf for all the time and manifold efforts in organizing, processing and refining all 11 chapters of this impressive book. I sincerely thank all of the internationally renowned authors who contributed highly informative manuscripts. As always, the precise and fast copy editing work of Martina Guttenbach is highly appreciated. The constant interest in and support of *Monographs in Human Genetics* by the publisher, Thomas Karger, motivates us to continue with this timely book series.

Michael Schmid, Würzburg

Preface

The earliest descriptions of hearing loss appear in the Edwin Smith Surgical Papyrus, the oldest known scientific document dating around 3,000 BC. The Papyrus described how temporal bone trauma and basilar skull fractures affected the hearing and speech in those wounded from battles and remarkably suggested there were even physicians specializing only in the ears. The advancement of medicine, with no exception to otology, witnessed a painfully slow evolution throughout the following centuries, and the birth of genetics would not happen until the 19th century.

Millennia later, after the emergence of modern genetics and arrival of the post-genomics era, in stark contrast to the initial descriptions of trauma-related hearing loss, it is clear that genetics is responsible for the majority of all hearing loss. As conventional genomics approaches have once again shifted, this time in favour of high-throughput sequencing, the genetics community is once again witness to a surge of data. With the availability of the fully annotated human genome, it seems the next great endeavour is annotating the variants in the human genome and understanding their underlying molecular mechanisms. We also find ourselves on the dawn of a precision medicine movement that will be heavily directed by genetics discoveries of past and present. One could assert that there has never been a more exciting time to be engaged in scientific research, more specifically auditory science research, than today.

Perhaps it is the unparalleled layers of heterogeneity epitomizing hereditary hearing loss so well or even the sheer complexity of the auditory system and its impact on language acquisition and social development that makes this such an intriguing field. Quickly developing technologies have allowed us thus far to probe questions our scientific predecessors have only envisaged. Given that hereditary hearing loss is the most common sensory deficit, major milestones have the potential to impact countless individuals.

This 20th volume of *Monographs in Human Genetics* is dedicated to the genetics of hearing loss. Our inspiration for its conception is to bring attention to a multifactorial and complex condition with prevalence greater than that of even Down syndrome that is oftentimes neither openly discussed nor diagnosed quickly enough and associated with ageism and other negative stereotypes. In an ever-increasing and ageing population, hearing health should be prioritized across the lifespan, as hearing loss has many broad indirect effects on the individual and society. Although it is truly impossible to cover all aspects of hearing loss genetics in a single monograph, we hope it will serve as an informative reference to showcase some of its appreciable diversity. This monograph intends to provide insight into several divergent but interconnected topics that could only be accomplished through the gracious contributions of an outstanding collection of international researchers who have dedicated much of their careers to addressing many of the fundamental issues in auditory science.

The monograph opens with a truly intimate insider's perspective of the deaf community from three remarkable women, all of whom are accomplished academics, who view their deafness as an integral part to their overall self-constructions. The next chapter recounts the broader impact of hearing loss, particularly in relation to age-related hearing loss and its social and psychological consequences. Then the monograph transitions toward diagnostic-oriented approaches by presenting two chapters describing how comprehensive genomics data in combination with regular audiological assessment and newborn hearing screening facilitate a precise and early diagnosis. An update of the current challenges and future directions of making a diagnosis as well as the genetics of nonsyndromic deafness and modifiers of hearing loss are presented in the following chapters. The subsequent two chapters highlight age-related hearing loss and its genetic modifiers in mice, continuing with a chapter describing the utility zebrafish provide in modelling deafness and their potential role in regenerative strategies. Finally, the monograph ends with a chapter about cochlear gene therapy and spiral ganglion neuronal preservation and regeneration.

We extend our gratitude to Karger Publishers and the Series Editor Michael Schmid for providing a platform for some of the brightest minds of the field to share their insight and draw attention to a worthy subject. We are humbled by the positive responses of the contributing authors and thankful for their valuable time. This monograph was composed for clinicians, researchers, and students with the aim of providing inspirational and stimulating insight into such an exciting field. We graciously thank Dr. Indrajit Nanda for valuable advice throughout the assembly of this book. Last but not least, we thank the patients and their families for their generous contributions to the field, to whom we are all profoundly indebted.

Barbara Vona, Würzburg
Thomas Haaf, Würzburg

Vona B, Haaf T (eds): Genetics of Deafness. Monogr Hum Genet. Basel, Karger, 2016, vol 20, pp 1–8
(DOI: 10.1159/000442334)

Genetics and Deafness: A View from the Inside

Teresa Blankmeyer Burke[a] · Kristin Snoddon[b] · Erin Wilkinson[c]

[a]Department of Philosophy, Gallaudet University, Washington, D.C., USA; [b]School of Linguistics and Language Studies, Carleton University, Ottawa, Ont., and [c]Department of Linguistics, University of Manitoba, Winnipeg, Man., Canada

Abstract

This chapter presents a cross-disciplinary overview of genetics and deafness from the perspective of 3 deaf academics employed in tenured or tenure-track positions at American and Canadian universities. We present a collective examination of the science of genetics and deafness using perspectives gained through disciplinary-specific research in bioethics, deaf and disability studies, education, linguistics, and philosophy. Specifically, we analyze the relationship between genetic patterning and language diversity, and then move to an analysis of bioethical issues related to deaf people and social policy.

© 2016 S. Karger AG, Basel

This chapter presents a cross-disciplinary overview of genetics and deafness from the perspective of 3 deaf academics employed in tenured or tenure-track positions at American and Canadian universities. In surveying how deaf people are positioned within broader discourses of genetics and medical science, we present our individual experiences of deaf culture and community, and how our bodies of research are respectively informed by this existence.

The chapter begins with a brief biography and introduction of each author's field of specialization as it engages with communities of deaf and signed language peoples. We then present a collective examination of the science of genetics and deafness using perspectives gained through disciplinary-specific research in bioethics, deaf and disability studies, education, linguistics, and philosophy. Specifically, the chapter begins by positioning the relationship between genetic patterning and language diversity, and then moves to a consideration of bioethical issues related to deaf people and social policy.

Background

Rather than describing deaf culture as an abstract, monolithic entity, we recognize that narrations of our diverse lived experiences of deaf culture and community may be the most effective means of presenting deaf ways of being in the world.

Teresa Blankmeyer Burke is a professor of Philosophy at Gallaudet University. She grew up in a hearing family in the suburbs of Los Angeles, and received a mainstream primary and secondary education with no support other than her hearing aids. As a teenager, she began learning signed language, using note-taking services in college and moving to signed language interpreters in graduate school.

Kristin Snoddon is a professor of Applied Linguistics and Discourse Studies at Carleton University, Canada. She grew up in a hearing family in small-town Ontario and was deafened at the age of 5 by spinal meningitis. She did not learn signed language until she was 21 and in her last year of undergraduate studies at the University of Toronto.

Erin Wilkinson is a professor of Linguistics at the University of Manitoba in Canada. She was born to a hearing family in the late 1970s and grew up in Kansas City, a large midwestern city in the United States. Thanks to an ongoing large-scale study on Connexin 26 at Gallaudet University in Washington, D.C., she learned that the cause of her deafness was the recessive gene of Connexin 26. Her primary, secondary, and post-secondary education were primarily facilitated through signed language interpreters, except for when she received direct communication with teachers when she was a foreign exchange student at a deaf boarding school in Norway and at Gallaudet University for her Masters degree.

The 3 authors' brief biographies illustrate diverse etiologies and types of hearing loss, bilingual language learning profiles, and the varying access to educational supports available in urban versus rural settings. For each of us, deafness is an integral and necessary part of our respective self-constructions, and should not be adduced as tragedy, barrier or obstacle to human flourishing. In this way, we are collectively representative of the diverse deaf communities described in this paper. Related to this, the next section discusses the relationship between genetics and signed language communities.

The Role of Recessive Genes in Transmission and Maintenance of Signed Languages

Around the world, linguists are studying signed languages to not only learn more about their linguistic structures but also how they fit into the big picture of the definition of human languages. Signed language research provides crucial pieces to the puzzle of language genesis and evolution. This is due to the unique development of signed languages, as their evolutionary development is much shorter and more precarious than spoken languages, and they are at a higher risk of endangerment. For instance, Nonaka [1] describes the prevalent cycle of signed language development where signed languages are 'quickly created then stabilized for a brief period, then die', exemplifying one typical characteristic of signed languages. The transmission and maintenance of signed languages appear to be dependent on genetic patterning of 2 types of signed language communities since genetic patterning is partially responsible for the spread (and endangerment) of signed languages [2]. In a broader sense, investigating signed languages and their community members leads researchers to observe the factors lent to language transmission and maintenance.

However, it would be inaccurate to view genetic factors as the sole origin of deaf populations. For instance, deafness is the most commonly reported disability in Nigeria, where over 10 million people are reported to be deaf or hard of hearing [3]. In this context, childhood illnesses associated with poverty contribute to the statistically high rate of deafness [4]. The World Federation of the Deaf states that 80% of the world's deaf people live in developing countries, where environmental factors apart from genetics similarly contribute to the creation and maintenance of deaf populations [5]. These environmental factors have become less prevalent in Western contexts with better access to health care and vaccinations [6].

Signed languages are categorized by their sociocultural and linguistic characteristics, and their users are identified as belonging to either sign language macro-communities or sign language micro-communities [7]. Sign language macro-communities are predominately found in industrialized countries and in urban communities, such as those found in Brazil and the United States. Historically, residential schools for the deaf in these countries served to bring together numerous deaf children from different parts of the country and introduce these children to signed language. Deaf children in these contexts most often acquire their signed language from deaf adults and peers at residential schools rather than from their families, thereby exemplifying atypical language transmission. Sign language macro-communities are generally stable, since there are large communities of deaf signers along with deaf schools to maintain signed languages.

In sign language macro-communities, deaf people actively seek (unrelated) deaf partners to raise families; this is the cultural practice of non-random or assortative mating. An increase in the deaf-deaf mating pattern would increase the number of carriers of Connexin 26 recessive genes as this mutation is very common among people who are born deaf, and arguably may lead to group consciousness as they identify themselves as unique and separate from hearing people [8].

Sign language micro-communities are described as small, labor-economy-based communities where mixed hearing and deaf marriages are the norm. The prevalence of recessive genes in micro-communities is much higher than it is in macro-communities, and also 'the relatively high birth rates might affect early language acquisition, as they result in more older signing siblings, more carriers and more deaf family members in overlapping generations' [2]. Unlike macro-communities, in micro-communities hearing signers play a critical role in signed language transmission and maintenance.

Genetic patterning as well as societal oppression predicts the type of linguistic and social structures, such as marriage practices, that occur in signed language communities. If the environment is predominantly deaf with few hearing members, and if the majority does not encourage equity for deaf people in employment and educational opportunities, then it is suggested that deaf people perceive themselves as a separate group from hearing people and actively seek deaf partners to raise families. If the environment is highly mixed, consisting of deaf and hearing members, then deaf people will not have a group identity that separates them from hearing members and will not actively seek deaf partners. Instead, they will seek partners who share the same linguistic and cultural practices [8]. A historical genetic study of 3 communities in the northeastern United States indicates that language use is interrelated with deaf genetic patterning, along with marriage practices and consciousness of a group consisting only of deaf members [8]. Both deaf-deaf and mixed deaf-hearing mating patterns suggest that the ability to sign, rather than deaf status, is the main motivation behind partner selection [2].

However, the issue of deaf intermarriage contributing to deaf populations has been contentious since Bell first published his work in 1883 [9] advocating deaf-focused eugenic practices, which included sterilization and a recommended ban on deaf-deaf marriages [10]. In a United States context, only 5–8% of deaf children are born to deaf parents [11]. In spite of this, deaf people are stated to have one of the highest rates of endogamous marriage of any ethnic group; Ladd places this figure at 90% [12]. Kusters also reports that micro-communities can vary in terms of deaf people's pairing with deaf or hearing partners, with cultural and educational factors suggested as possible contributors [13].

Genetic patterning in signed language communities has several outcomes. There will be a growth in the hereditary deaf population. The increased incidence of recessive deafness in both macro- and micro-communities leads to more stability in language transmission and maintenance of community signed languages [2].

In order to illustrate how particular sociocultural features frame perspectives on deafness, the following example is provided regarding a Balinese village known for a high incidence of recessive deafness.

Sociocultural Construction of Deafness: Actual Example

De Vos describes the sociocultural construction of deafness in an isolated village called Desa Kolok in Bali, Indonesia [14]. Deaf villagers are fully integrated in all aspects of community life in its social, economical, religious, and political functions; this is strikingly different from other societies where deaf people find themselves marginalized and struggle to assimilate. Deaf villagers in Desa Kolok have special roles in arts and employment where they perform deaf dances and martial arts, and work on water line maintenance and as gravediggers. Both deaf and hearing villagers believe in a deaf god [14]. This example of a sign language micro-community serves in part to illustrate how the cultural meanings of deafness are constructed in different contexts. However, as occurs in other contexts, current social policies concerning deaf people are changing both the cultural positioning of deaf individuals as a group and the genetic patterns that contribute to various deaf communities.

Consequences of Changes in the Recessive Gene Pool

To date, some sign language micro-communities including the Al-Sayyid Bedouins and Desa Kolok are beginning to experience changes in their social and cultural practices. Deaf children in these communities are being sent to boarding schools far from their villages where the children are introduced to unrelated deaf populations and different signed language varieties. Employment is another motivation for deaf people to migrate outside of their home communities. Given higher mobility in education and employment, there appears to be a gradual divergence between deaf and hearing community members, and their marriage practices are changing as deaf people seek deaf partners outside of their sociocultural/linguistic home community. This will predictably result in a shift in genetic patterning, as there will be fewer mixed deaf-hearing marriages. Not only will this result in a decreased incidence of deafness and of hearing community members who share a signed language, it also predicts the potential death of indigenous signed languages, as future generations will experience different social and cultural practices from the previous generations [15, 16]. In this way, sign language micro-communities may appear to dissolve into structures that bear resemblance to sign language macro-communities.

The Pervasiveness of Signing Deaf Communities

Despite the threat of language death in the sign language micro-communities described above, and the reduction in deaf populations suggested by genetic technology, signing deaf communities have proven to be surprisingly resilient. In a Western context, factors contributing to deaf cultural maintenance include the tendency for deaf children and youth to be placed in signing programs after having been deemed as failing in mainstream environments which lack access to signed language [17]. More positively, deaf adolescents and young adults (including those with milder hearing losses) tend to seek out opportunities to learn signed language and participate in deaf communities [18]. As Breda Carty notes, 'the number of signers of interest to linguists is not necessarily the same as the number of Deaf people who … regard the language as important in their social and cultural lives' [18]. Included in the latter group may be the deaf children of hearing parents who seek to learn signed language. The second author's current study investigates the development of intensive signed language curricula for meeting the learning needs of hearing parents in the Netherlands and Canada; parental demand for this type of program appears to be unprecedented [19]. Nearly all parent participants report having children who use cochlear implants.

Similarly, signed language classes for second language (hearing) learners remain robust course offerings at postsecondary institutions around the world. In February 2015, the Modern Language Association reported that American Sign Language enrollments had increased by 216% at the graduate level [20]. The success of learning any second language is often dependent on opportunities to use the language in context; thus, it might be hoped that postsecondary signed language learners will seek out deaf communities to extend their learning experience. In sum, the resilience of deaf people as a group and the continued cultural interest in signed languages may be strong enough to survive technological forays into genetic terrain and other social policies that deliberately or incidentally target the existence of signed language communities. The next section of the paper discusses in depth some bioethical dimensions of genetic research and technology related to deaf people.

The Chicken-Egg Problem: Eradication, Are We Eradicating Deafness or Deaf People?

The previous sections of this paper provided an overview of signed language communities and biographical vignettes of the authors' lives, which by many, if not most, accounts would be viewed as successful, productive human lives regardless of hearing status. There is a potential risk with such accounts, since it leaves open the objection that we represent only a certain segment of deaf people, and that the authors' lives are the exception, not the rule, to what deaf lives are typically imagined to be like. This perception has its basis

in pervasive barriers to education and employment that are faced by deaf people around the world and that are perpetuated by social policies affecting this population. Medical interventions for deaf children are focused on restoring hearing as a means of preventing delayed language development; however, the efficacy of cochlear implants in supporting first-language acquisition in congenitally deaf children is limited [21]. Frequently, these interventions are accompanied by policy restrictions on signed language learning despite evidence for the benefits that learning signed language provides for deaf and hard of hearing children's development [22]. This relates to an important set of questions that drive discussion about ethical uses of genetic research, development and technology in bioethics and philosophy, which is the focus of this section.

We begin with 2 philosophical puzzles. The first puzzle, call this the Pursuit of Science puzzle, asks whether one ought to pursue genetic research on deafness with the aim of eradicating deafness, given that such a pursuit might have the secondary effect of drastically reducing, or even eradicating the class of sociolinguistic communities that use a signed language. This puzzle is further complicated by the claims of linguists, who argue that research on communities of signed language users can provide important information.

Technology derived from genetic research such as preimplantation genetic diagnosis (PGD)[1] and noninvasive prenatal diagnosis (NIPD) has the potential to drastically impact the number of

[1] Preimplantation genetic diagnosis (PGD) involves genetic screening of fertilized eggs that result as products of in vitro fertilization (IVF). This screening occurs before the fertilized egg is implanted in the uterus. In most cases, genetic screening is done to rule out undesired genetic or chromosomal variation. Noninvasive prenatal diagnosis (NIPD) occurs after pregnancy is established (usually, non IVF precipitated pregnancy) and is conducted through a simple blood test of the pregnant woman. The fetal genetic profile is constructed from fragments of fetal DNA present in the pregnant woman's blood sample.

deaf infants that are born, at least in developed nations where such technology is readily available[2]. Of course, genetic heritage is not the only means by which people become deaf[3], but the age of onset and the impact this has on language acquisition and choice of language is relevant to the flourishing of signed language communities, given the importance of a critical mass of native language users [6]. While it has been observed that most deaf individuals will acquire a signed language and thereby join this sociolinguistic community [18, 23], the case of already existing deaf people is different from the case of potential deaf people who do not get to exist.

The genetic profiling of embryos before implantation that occurs in PGD offers potential parents a choice – they may opt to implant embryos that have tested positive for characteristics such as deafness, or they may opt against implanting such embryos. When an embryo that possesses the characteristic of deafness is *not* selected for implantation, the question then becomes whether that decision is ethically justifiable. Since ethical decision-making often weighs considerations of harm, one way to assess this is by asking whether an entity that does not get to exist can be harmed [24]. The person-affecting account of harm assumes that harm is something that must affect a person or future person; the claim here is that the (deaf) embryo that was not selected has not been harmed because it is not a person.

Consider now a different outcome, in which the deaf embryo *is* selected. Even if deafness is a person-affecting harm (which is an open question), has the deaf embryo been harmed by being brought into existence? Note that this is not a matter of a particular potential person being born deaf or hearing, but a matter of choosing one potential person over the other. On this account, in order to claim that the deaf future person has been harmed, one must maintain that the harm of deafness outweighs the benefit of existence. This culminates in the Non-Identity Problem puzzle, which asks whether existence-inducing choices can be harmful, even when they appear to be bad for no one [24].

Taken together, the Non-Identity Problem puzzle and the Pursuit of Science puzzle offer a series of ethical questions for those who engage in genetics research on deafness: Does research on genetics harm deaf persons or future deaf persons? Does genetic technology harm future members of signed language communities? Should there be constraints on genetic selection for or against deafness? Is there a moral duty to select for or against deafness? Is it ethically better to choose a hearing embryo over a deaf embryo?

These questions rest on fundamental assumptions about wellbeing, value, and meaning, or what components constitute a flourishing human life. Views about these components come into play for potential parents making choices about whether to continue or terminate a pregnancy, and particularly if the embryo or fetus has features that are not species-typical. Potential parents may find it difficult to imagine a deaf child with a flourishing life, not distinguishing between the importance of access to language, access to environmental sounds, and access to aesthetic sounds [25]. Researchers may disassociate themselves from the potential consequences of their work, reasoning that even when bench science

---

[2] At the time of this writing, use of NIPD (also referred to as noninvasive prenatal testing) is still restricted to a certain set of genetic conditions. At this time, genetic deafness is not one of those conditions, though research is currently underway on this. See Meng et al. [28] who consider the testing for *GJB2*.

[3] Widespread outbreaks of disease have contributed to rates of deafness in a population; the 'rubella bulge' of more than 8,000 deaf children born between 1963–1965 is a particular instance of this [29]. With the advent of immunizations for diseases associated with deafness (including rubella, measles, mumps, bacterial meningitis, chicken pox), this may generate less of an effect than during the preimmunization era. Still, some diseases known to cause prenatal deafness such as herpes and cytomegalovirus do not yet have effective vaccines.

results in clinical applications, the proximate cause is parental decision-making, not scientific knowledge gains.

Finally, if the potential for eradication of a community rests on individual parental choice in a liberal society where parents are given autonomous choice in reproductive decision-making, this pits a tradition of parental autonomy against group claims for preservation. One way to frame this is by appealing to moral notions of rights, but this is tricky, since rights by traditional definition attach to individuals and not groups [26]. Group rights are defined as rights that attach to the group, not the rights claims of individual members of a group in virtue of their status as members of the group. Cultural and linguistic groups have asserted moral claims that their culture and language ought to be respected and protections accorded in the public domain, with these protections secured by law. However, this presents another puzzle, since it raises the question of how far a state ought to go to preserve a cultural and linguistic community – does the state's responsibility to preserve and protect a minority community extend to limiting rights of procreative freedom?

To this point, the United Nations' first international human rights treaty of the 21st century, the Convention on the Rights of Persons with Disabilities (CRPD), explicitly outlines measures for states to take regarding the promotion of signed languages and the linguistic identity of the deaf community in the education system and beyond. Signed language rights for deaf children straddle the divide between language rights (which are collective rights) and disability rights, which are typically cast by national legislation as individual rights to access. The CRPD's framing of signed language rights aligns with how Skutnabb-Kangas and Phillipson describe linguistic human rights as encompassing the right to identify with a mother tongue and receive educa-tion and public services in that language [27]. With its explicit adoption of a social model of disability, the CRPD maintains disability as a social and political identity. Thus, this treaty outlines protections for deaf people as a group (including deaf infants and children and those concerned with their welfare).

The puzzles offered above provide 3 different vantage points from which to consider the impact and implications of applications of genetic technology: those of the parent, the scientist, and society. The analysis of the views operates on a thin conception of deaf life that is insufficiently robust for determining the social conditions that contribute to a flourishing deaf life. As indicated earlier in this paper, deaf people demonstrate affinities for joining signed language communities that suggest these should be a main consideration. In our idiosyncratic ways, the authors of this paper have chosen to live our lives as part of the deaf communities in our midst. Thus, our academic views of genetics and deafness are necessarily tied to these values.

Conclusion

In our chapter, we have attempted to highlight several issues regarding the relationship between genetic patterning and various types of signed language communities, as well as bioethical questions that emerge with the development of genetic technologies. We have also attempted to show how worldwide cultural conceptions of what it means to be a deaf individual constitute and are constituted by social policies which in turn affect signed language communities and genetic patterning. It is our hope that our narration of these issues 'from the inside' will serve to illuminate and inform the work of geneticists in terms of seeking clarification of goals for the human project.

References

1 Nonaka AM: Sign languages – the forgotten endangered languages: lessons on the importance of remembering. Lang Soc 2004;33:737–767.

2 Gialluisi A, Dediu D, Francks C, Fisher SE: Persistence and transmission of recessive deafness and sign language: new insights from village sign languages. Eur J Hum Genet 2013;21:894–896.

3 Ajavon P: A sign language for Nigeria; in Commonwealth Education Partnerships 2011:37. http://www.cedol.org/wp-content/uploads/2012/02/Paulina-Ajavon-article.pdf.

4 Eleweke CJ: A review of issues in deaf education under Nigeria's 6-3-3-4 education system. J Deaf Stud Deaf Educ 2002;7:74–82.

5 World Federation of the Deaf: Human rights. http://wfdeaf.org/human-rights (accessed March 3, 2015).

6 Johnston T: W(h)ither the deaf community? Population, genetics and the future of Australian sign language. Am Ann Deaf 2004;148:358–375.

7 Fenlon J, Wilkinson E: Sign languages in the world; in Schembri A, Lucas C (eds): Sociolinguistics and Deaf Communities. Cambridge, Cambridge University Press, 2015, pp 5–28.

8 Lane H, Pillard RC, French M: Origins of the American deaf-world: assimilating and differentiating societies and their relation to genetic patterning. Sign Lang Studies 2000;1:17–44.

9 Bell AG: Upon the formation of a deaf variety of the human race. Nat Acad Sci Mem 1883;2:177–262.

10 Lane H: Ethnicity, ethics, and the Deaf-World. J Deaf Stud Deaf Educ 2005;10:291–310.

11 Mitchell RE, Karchmer MA: Chasing the mythical ten percent: parental status of deaf and hard of hearing students in the United States. Sign Lang Studies 2004;4:138–163.

12 Ladd P: Understanding Deaf Culture: In Search of Deafhood. North York, Multilingual Matters, 2003.

13 Kusters A: Deaf utopias? Reviewing the sociocultural literature on the world's 'Martha's Vineyard Situations'. J Deaf Stud Deaf Educ 2010;15:3–16.

14 De Vos C: A signers' village in Bali, Indonesia. Minpaku Anthropol Newsl 2011;33:4–5.

15 Kisch S: Demarcating generations of signers in the dynamic sociolinguistic landscape of a shared sign language: the case of the Al-Sayyid Bedouin; in Zeshan U, de Vos C (eds): Sign Languages in Village Communities: Anthropological and Linguistic Insights. Nijmegen, Ishara Press, 2012, pp 87–126.

16 Padden C: Sign language geography; in Mathur G, Napoli DJ (eds): Deaf Around the World. New York, Oxford University Press, 2011, pp 19–37.

17 Akamatsu C, Musselman C, Zwiebel A: Nature versus nurture in the development of cognition in deaf people; in Spencer PE, Erting CJ, Marschark M (eds): The Deaf Child in the Family and the School: Essays in Honour of Kathryn P. Meadow-Orlans. Mahwah, Lawrence Erlbaum Associates, 2000, pp 255–274.

18 Carty B: Comments on 'W(h)ither the Deaf community?' Sign Lang Studies 2006;6:181–189.

19 Snoddon K: Using the *Common European Framework of Reference for Languages* to teach sign language to parents of deaf children. CMLR/RCLV 2015;71:270–287.

20 Goldberg D, Looney D, Lusin N: Enrollments in languages other than English in United States institutions of higher education, fall 2013. New York, Modern Language Association of America, 2015. www.mla.org/pdf/2013_enrollment_survey.pdf (accessed February 26, 2015).

21 Humphries T, Kushalnagar P, Mathur G, Napoli DJ, Padden C, et al: Language acquisition for deaf children: reducing the harms of zero tolerance to the use of alternative approaches. Harm Reduction J 2012;9:16.

22 Snoddon K: American Sign Language and early intervention. Can Mod Lang Rev 2008;64:581–604.

23 Piñar P, Dussias PE, Morford JP: Deaf readers as bilinguals: an examination of deaf readers' print comprehension in light of current advances in bilingualism and second language progressing. Lang Linguist Compass 2011;5:691–704.

24 Parfit D: Reasons and Persons. Oxford, Clarendon Press, 1987.

25 Burke TB: The Quest for a Deaf Child: Ethics and Genetics. Unpublished Doctoral Dissertation, University of New Mexico, 2011.

26 Wenar L: Rights; in Zalta E (ed): The Stanford Encyclopedia of Philosophy, Fall 2011. Stanford, Stanford University, 2011. http://plato.stanford.edu/archives/fall2011/entries/rights/.

27 Skutnabb-Kangas T, Phillipson R: Linguistic human rights, past and present; in Skutnabb-Kangas T, Phillipson R (eds): Linguistic Human Rights: Overcoming Linguistic Discrimination. Berlin, Mouton de Gruyter, 1995, pp 71–110.

28 Meng M, Li X, Ge H, Chen F, Han M, et al: Noninvasive prenatal testing for autosomal recessive conditions by maternal plasma sequencing in a case of congenital deafness. Genet Med 2014;12:972–976.

29 Karmel CK: 'Rubella bulge' of the 60's reaches the colleges. New York Times, April 25, 1982. http://www.nytimes.com/1982/04/25/education/rubella-bulge-of-the-60-s-reaches-the-colleges.html.

Erin Wilkinson, PhD
Department of Linguistics, University of Manitoba
536 Fletcher Argue Building
Winnipeg, MB, R3T 5V5 (Canada)
E-Mail Erin.Wilkinson@umanitoba.ca

Vona B, Haaf T (eds): Genetics of Deafness. Monogr Hum Genet. Basel, Karger, 2016, vol 20, pp 9–18
(DOI: 10.1159/000444561)

Hearing Loss in Older Age and Its Effect on the Individuals, Their Families and the Community

Catherine M. McMahon

Department of Linguistics, Macquarie University, Sydney, N.S.W., and HEARing Co-operative Research Centre, Melbourne, Vic.,
Australia

Abstract

Relationships are central to social well-being and emotional resilience across the lifespan, and good hearing and communication is integral to their establishment and maintenance. However, hearing loss is one of the most prevalent chronic conditions of ageing and significantly affects communication. Age-related hearing loss (ARHL), also known as presbycusis, typically is slowly progressive and commonly managed many years after being identified, increasing the risk of social withdrawal, early retirement, depression and mortality, and other negative consequences. ARHL occurs as the combination of environmental exposures, vascular insults, trauma, genetic predisposition, and metabolic changes. Further, it is associated with other age-related medical and health conditions, such as falls and dementia, although the relationship between these remains unclear. Despite multiple studies reporting that hearing devices are associated with positive outcomes in speech, communication and quality of life measures, the uptake and use of these is relatively low in many countries. As hearing loss is expected to rise with the ageing population, it is considered a major public health problem that needs to be addressed in the near future. © 2016 S. Karger AG, Basel

Age-related hearing loss (ARHL) is a highly prevalent yet relatively poorly addressed public health problem in the older population, which affects them, their families and the community [1–5]. According to the World Health Organization (WHO), ~360 million people worldwide have significant (or disabling) hearing loss, classified as >40 dB hearing level (HL) pure tone average hearing thresholds at octave frequencies between 0.5 Hz to 4 kHz [6]. Further, approximately one-third of people >65 years of age are affected by significant hearing loss, which increases with advancing age and is most prevalent in low- and middle-income countries [7] or in areas of socio-economic disadvantage within higher-income countries [8]. The prevalence increases as milder forms of hearing loss are included, where the most commonly used definition in the literature is a pure tone average loss ≥25 dB HL. Even in middle-aged adults (between 45–60 years), using this more common definition of hearing loss in the better ear, the prevalence of hearing loss in the UK is ~10% [9].

Given the ageing demographic, increasing average life span, and risks to hearing from recreational noise exposure (e.g. from personal audio devices), chronic hearing loss is projected to significantly increase [10]. Genetic forms of hearing loss certainly contribute to ARHL [11], and twin studies suggest that they may account for approximately half of the variance in the population with environmental factors accounting for the rest [12, 13]. However, because of the variability in the onset, magnitude and change in hearing loss over time, genetic factors become increasingly difficult to differentiate from other causes. Disruptions to the same gene can result in different magnitudes and configurations of hearing loss, and interactions between environmental insults and genetics vary across individuals. Therefore, specific genetic markers are yet unclear, although mouse models of ageing yield promising results for the future [14].

Because hearing loss is gradual in nature in most individuals, it is typically diagnosed and managed several years after its onset [15], often after having led to multiple negative consequences. These include reduced employment, poor quality of life, social isolation, depressive symptoms, somatic symptoms, and increased mortality risk [16–19]. As hearing loss interferes with so many of life's activities, it may prove to be a major impediment to society's need to have people remain longer in the workforce as the proportion of 'working age' people in developed countries shrinks [20]. Due to workplace separation and early retirement from hearing loss as well as direct and indirect medical costs, the economic cost of hearing loss is high; estimated to be about 2–3%

of the gross national product in the USA and about 1.4% of the gross national income in Australia [21, 22].

Despite hearing loss being considered a major public health problem, multiple barriers exist to seeking hearing healthcare, even in higher income countries where hearing healthcare is often partly or fully funded by national healthcare schemes. One of the most commonly cited barriers for accessing hearing healthcare, other than perceived need and cost, is the stigma associated with hearing aids and ageism [23]. Yet, this is often not addressed within rehabilitation programs. Traditional models of hearing healthcare use a biomedical framework. In such cases, hearing loss is managed in isolation from other age-related sensory and cognitive declines, and the impairment itself is the focus of diagnosis and management, rather than identifying solutions for the handicapping effects of hearing loss or the stigma associated with this. Therefore, hearing devices are often a major focus of the solution rather than a part of managing the disability it creates [24]. On the other hand, as hearing loss is a chronic problem, then rehabilitative models should consider the individuals within a bio-psycho-social and environmental framework. In particular, the International Classification of Functioning, Disability and Health (ICF, http://psychiatr.ru/download/1313?view=1&name=ICF_18.pdf) provides a framework that considers the pathophysiology of the hearing loss (body), its effect on speech understanding and comprehension (activity), and its effect on the individual's ability to participate in social, educational and occupational activities (participation). It also considers the influence of the environment (e.g. whether it impedes communication with excessive noise) and the person (such as their psychological or emotional state). Recent literature certainly encourages audiologists to use such an approach in the management of individuals with hearing loss (e.g. [25]).

For rehabilitation programs of ARHL to be successful, these should broadly consider the effect of hearing loss and its consequences on successful ageing. Life course perspectives, such as the life course health development model, encourage an ecological view which is inclusive of multiple biological, psychological and social factors that combine to produce health [26]. Consequently, the relationship between hearing ability and successful ageing is the result of multiple interacting factors over a person's lifetime and an individual's ability to adapt to this. The combined effects of ageing and noise and ototoxic substance exposure sustained across the life course remain key factors in the development of hearing loss into adulthood [27, 28]. However, it is likely that these are modulated by genetic and other sociodemographic factors, including access to healthcare services, which may change over time. Therefore, 2 individuals who have similar environmental and occupational exposures might have very different audiometric profiles; and those with similar audiometric profiles may perceive very different magnitudes of disability and handicap.

Reconceptualising hearing loss within a broader model of health and ageing would enable more effective solutions to be devised and implemented that could include: more effective management of the individuals with hearing loss and their significant others that considers not only the hearing loss but also other age-related declines that affect communication and social participation; implementation of legislation and policies that reduce exposure to loud noise and ototoxic substances; and creation of more accessible environments that minimise the handicapping effects of hearing loss and other age-related declines.

Risk Factors for ARHL

One of the best documented risks of hearing loss in middle/older age is exposure to loud noise. A recent bulletin from the WHO estimates that 1.1 billion people worldwide might be at risk of developing noise-induced hearing loss [29]. Occupational noise is estimated to account for ~16% of all hearing loss worldwide (ranging from 7–21%), yet is preventable [30]. Recommended exposure standards and regulations exist in many countries, but there is difficulty in their implementation, both practically and politically. This is highlighted in a recent Cochrane systematic review of 25 studies assessing the effectiveness of interventions to reduce occupational noise exposure or hearing loss [31]. Of these, 1 study showed that legislation could lead to a measureable reduction in noise exposure levels at a local level. However, very low-quality evidence across 4 of these studies showed that effective use of hearing protection devices is associated with less hearing loss than poorer use of hearing protection devices, and there is no evidence that hearing protection programs reduce the risk of hearing loss to levels equivalent to non-exposed workers. Further, growing concerns exist over noise exposure in young adults via personal music systems, night clubs and live music events. A study of 356 young adults in the UK in 2000 shows that, while the risk of occupational noise exposure has reduced since the early 1980s, the risk of social noise exposure has tripled [32]. While reports on the effect of exposure on hearing thresholds vary, more recent evidence in animals suggests that subclinical damage may exist [33] that affects their ability to hear, particularly in more challenging listening situations. Research suggests that loud noise exposure affects the high-threshold neurons of the cochlea, so that while pure tone thresholds themselves may recover after an exposure preserving normal audiometric thresholds, the dynamic range is significantly and permanently affected [34]. Additionally, prolonged exposure to environmental noise, even at 'safe' exposure levels <80 dB(A), causes non-auditory effects on health, including headaches, increased stress and fatigue in adults, consistent with the increases in catecholamine and cortical levels seen in animal models (for a review, see [35]). As reviewed in Basner et al. [17], population-based studies have shown that high levels of noise exposure, whether occupational or environmental (e.g. from road traffic or aircraft noise), are associated with increased risk of cardiovascular disease and mortality. There are few successful intervention programs that address both occupational and recreational exposure to loud noise, and certainly most do not take into account the effects of loud noise on the broader aspects of health.

Other known risks of ARHL include modifiable risk factors, such as smoking, nutrition, increased body mass index, and reduced exercise. For example, in the Blue Mountains Hearing Study, an Australian longitudinal study of hearing loss in 2,956 older adults (≥49 years of age), Gopinath et al. [36] showed that a higher mean glycaemic diet is a predictor of prevalent and incident hearing loss in older adults, increasing the risk of developing age-related hearing loss by 76%. Further, dietary intake of omega-3 in this population appears to confer a protective effect against ARHL, where consumption of ≥2 servings of fish per week reduced the risk by 46% compared with a dietary intake of <1 serving per week [37]. In another longitudinal population-based study of hearing loss in 3,753 older adults (≥48 years) conducted in the United States, the Epidemiology of Hearing Loss Study, it has been shown that cigarette smoking increases the risk of hearing loss, where current smokers were 1.69 times as likely to have a hearing loss as non-smokers (95% CI, 1.31–2.17) [5]. Further, those with increased risk of hearing loss included non-smokers who lived in the same household as current smokers. Importantly, these modifiable risks are not only associated with hearing loss, but also cognitive decline and mortality [38], suggesting that healthy and active lifestyles across the lifespan are important criteria for all aspects of successful ageing.

Ototoxic drugs have well-documented effects on cochlear and/or vestibular function, typically causing irreversible cellular damage, and include aminoglycoside antibiotics, platinum-based chemotherapeutic agents (cisplatin and carboplatin), loop diuretics, anti-malarial drugs, and salicylates [39]. At least in developed countries, these drugs are used for serious and/or life-threatening diseases so that the risks to health and function outweigh the risk of hearing loss [40]. However, in developing countries, the regulation and monitoring of drug prescription and over-the-counter provision is lacking, resulting in higher rates of hearing loss in younger adults. Nonetheless, even in developed countries, monitoring of auditory function is neither standard nor consistent [6]. Effective monitoring programs can reduce the magnitude of hearing loss through changes to the family of drugs administered, or the dosage. Further, these can also better prepare the individuals and their families how to manage the resultant hearing loss.

The susceptibility of an individual to ageing, noise and ototoxic substances is likely to be influenced or modified by his/her genetic make-up. Associations between family history and ARHL have been shown to exist across multiple population-based studies. For example, McMahon et al. [11] demonstrated that this association was strongest for more severe hearing loss, where a 3-fold increased risk was observed for women with a maternal history of hearing loss. Animal models of hearing loss support this, where specific strains of inbred mice are more likely to sustain hearing loss from ageing and noise trauma than others [41]. As well as genetic susceptibility, synergistic effects exist that increase the risk of hearing loss. While population-based cross-sectional studies have shown that cigarette smoking increases the risk of ARHL, even after excluding those with occupational noise exposure [5], several studies reported that smoking in working-age adults increases the risk of occupational hearing loss. Such risks presented in young to middle age presumably increase the risk and magnitude of hearing loss in later life. For example, Pouryaghoub et al. [42] evaluated the effect of smoking and noise exposure on hearing loss in 412 adult males working in a large food-producing factory, half who were self-reported smokers. They found statistically significant differences in the proportion of workers with hearing loss (using a 4-frequency average of 1, 2, 3, and 4 kHz >30 dB HL), where the risk of hearing loss for smokers was almost 8-fold. Using logistic regression analyses, they found significant associations with smoking, age and noise exposure duration. Synergistic effects between solvents and noise exposure, which commonly co-exist in industrial settings, have also been reported. Morata et al. [43] evaluated 124 noise-exposed workers who were also exposed to organic solvents and showed that age and toluene exposure (measured as hippuric acid), were significantly associated with hearing loss.

Behavioural and/or pharmacological interventions need to be implemented which are sustainable in the longer-term. For example, pharmacological prevention of hearing loss using glucocorticoids (such as dexamethasone) and/or neurotrophins (such as brain-derived neurotrophic factor) may be important in arresting the progression of cochlear hair-cell degeneration [44]. Further, behavioural interventions need to be implemented that are sensitive to the cultural diversity of the general public and which take a community-based approach to implementation.

Health-Related Associations with ARHL

There are a number of health-related problems that are associated with ARHL, including cognitive decline and self-reported falls, which both are independently associated with an increased risk of mortality [45, 46]. Probably the most notable association which has received considerable recent media attention is that between dementia and hearing loss [47–51]. In particular, using data from the Baltimore Longitudinal Study of Aging, a prospective longitudinal study of 639 older adults without dementia at baseline, Lin et al. [49]

showed that the hazard ratio of all-cause incident dementia for individuals with mild hearing loss was 1.89 (95% CI, 1.00–3.58) increasing to 4.94 (95% CI, 1.09–22.40) for those with severe hearing loss compared with those with normal hearing. While self-reported hearing aid use was not associated with a reduction in risk, hearing aid use and benefit were not measured within this study. Falls have also been related to ARHL, with a Finnish twin study of aging reporting an increase in the age-adjusted incidence rate ratio to 3.4 (95% CI, 1.0–11.4) in the poorest hearing quartiles compared to 1.2 (95% CI, 0.4–3.8) in the best hearing quartile [52]. In the US National Health and Nutritional Examination Survey, Lin and Ferrucci [53] also showed in adults between 40–69 years that for every 10-dB increase in hearing loss, there was a 1.4-fold (95% CI, 1.3–1.5) increased odds of reporting a fall over the preceding 12 months.

Lin and Ferrucci [53] proposed that these associations could be explained by different potential mechanisms, including: (1) a common neurobiological process where hearing loss, cognitive and physical declines could be associated with social or genetic factors not measured within current population-based studies; (2) a common neuropathologic process, which could include microvascular changes; or (3) a causal association where hearing loss causes increased cognitive load and sustained attention needed to process incoming information, or decreased social participation which may lead to degraded physical and cognitive capacity. Alternatively, such associations could also be driven by other common social determinants of health that were not assessed within the population-based studies [54]. Currently, several studies are being undertaken to further explore relationships between hearing loss, hearing aid use and cognitive and physical decline to determine whether hearing healthcare interventions might be successful in mitigating or reducing the effects of poor physical and cognitive health.

Barriers to Hearing Healthcare

Once a hearing loss does exist, rehabilitation interventions such as hearing aids appear to address many difficulties associated with impaired hearing [55]. Despite this, several studies indicate high levels of unmet need for hearing health services, poor use of prescribed hearing aids and, on average, a delay of 10 years prior to accessing hearing healthcare [24, 56]. While cost is often considered to be a barrier to the uptake of hearing aids, in fact similar prevalence rates of hearing aid uptake across countries with different hearing healthcare systems (i.e. a user pays system in the US vs. a government-funded system in the UK) exist. Importantly, evidence suggests that the later hearing rehabilitation occurs in the course of hearing loss, the less likely are older adults to continue to use and derive benefit from hearing aids [57]. Several studies have shown that help-seeking for hearing healthcare and the process of avoidance to acceptance of hearing aids is facilitated by perceived severity of hearing loss and its associated handicap. In a recent large-scale Australian study, major barriers to help-seeking for hearing loss and the successful use of hearing aids have been identified: negative attitudes to hearing aids, lack of support from family and low self-efficacy for hearing aid use [58, 59]. In addition, in a qualitative study of 10 first-time hearing aid users and 8 experienced hearing aid users, Wänström et al. [60] showed that hearing aid acceptance was facilitated by family support, accessibility of services and regular health assessments, but confounded by maladaptive coping mechanisms (such as withdrawal from communication opportunities) and stigma (typically associated with ageism). Several of these factors are rarely addressed within current models of hearing healthcare, limiting the access for those who live remotely and those who have less regular access to healthcare.

A systematic review has shown that the only predictor of hearing aid use is self-reported hearing difficulty [24]. It is assumed that as ARHL is associated with a slow decline in hearing, this may lead to over-accommodation of communication partners to speak loudly, and a gradual withdrawal from challenging listening situations that require mental effort to understand what is said. This, coupled with externalisation of the problem (e.g. 'other people mumble', see [61]), an acceptance of hearing loss as a part of natural ageing, and/or negative views on ageing, may interfere with the process of help-seeking. Addressing these barriers of readiness for treatment, family support and self-efficacy is essential to improve the outcomes of hearing healthcare for adults, and further work is necessary to develop and evaluate targeting interventions to address these key issues. Further, multiple studies have shown that general practitioners themselves pose a major barrier to accessing hearing healthcare (e.g. [62]), suggesting that the healthcare system itself needs to change to facilitate access for those with self-identified problems.

Current Hearing Healthcare Model Limits Choices and Access

Significant or disabling hearing loss is defined by the WHO as a pure tone average of octave frequencies between 0.5–4 kHz in the better ear >40 dB HL for adults [63]. However, the pure tone audiogram provides a measure of just-audible tones at different frequencies and speech understanding, limiting the ability to evaluate the impact of damage to the cochlea and auditory processing pathway on listening in everyday situations [34], which may be important for optimising the choice of technologies or signal-processing strategies. These tests are also insensitive to cochlear and auditory nerve damage that can occur through noise exposure, ageing and other factors before hearing thresholds become elevated. Furthermore, assessments are based on an evaluation of hearing alone and lack a holistic understanding of the individuals, their cognitive ability, perceived readiness for treatment and self-efficacy, all being important for the effective outcomes from hearing devices or other rehabilitation pathways. Typically, the solutions provided are device-focussed so the professional-client interaction is usually based around technology rather than motivation or ability to engage in a rehabilitative management program which can significantly influence their outcome [59]. While there is often a high level of hearing aid uptake and use reported for adults with more severe levels of hearing loss, this is typically not the case for milder forms of hearing loss, and the Blue Mountains Hearing Study showed that 42% of hearing devices fitted to older adults with mild hearing loss showed very low rates of usage of less than 1 hour per week [64]. In a recent systematic review, McCormack and Fortnum [65] reported that the most cited reasons given by participants not wearing hearing aids were a lack of perceived value/benefit provided by the hearing aid (particularly in noisy listening situations/background noise) and a lack of comfort. While hearing aids have substantially improved in technology over the years, they remain limited in their ability to improve speech in noisy environments. This may partly be due to a limitation in technology to overcome the damage to the auditory system, or due to unrealistic expectations of what their normal hearing peers are able to comprehend in complex listening environments due to other age-related declines.

A number of alternative interventions exist for individuals with hearing loss, including group or individual aural rehabilitation programs, counselling, supportive education, and assistive listening devices. Recent interest in the role of psychological therapies, such as motivational interviewing, is being explored within audiological settings to enhance the compliance with recommendations for management. However, audiologists are typically not provided with the skills to deliver this, and interdisciplinary management in healthcare for community-dwelling older adults remains rare.

Rehabilitation of ARHL and the Importance of Good Hearing Health

Hearing and communication are integral to successful ageing as they enable individuals to continue to function independently and maintain social relationships within the environments in which they live [66, 67]. Maintaining one's independence is associated with a better quality of life as a person ages, while maintenance of social relationships has been associated with better health and even reduced mortality among older adults [68]. It is assumed that better health results from the utilisation of social support networks during stressful conditions, as well as the reduction in cognitive decline, depression and other adverse emotional, behavioural and biological influences from regular social communication. Maintenance of good hearing, through minimising lifestyle risks of hearing loss, and good communication ability promotes independence so that older adults are less reliant on community services for everyday living requirements (meals, transport, etc.), which can also promote social interaction [69]. Good speech comprehension in adverse listening environments is facilitated by a combination of hearing, vision and cognition, each of which show declines with advancing age. Recently, there has been a renewed focus on understanding the interplay between these elements, particularly hearing and cognition [70], to develop remediation strategies that not only focus on the auditory input, but also address the cognitive processes that are needed to listen to the amplified (hearing aids) or vocoded (cochlear implants) sound signal. Nonetheless, with increasing age, the prevalence of co-morbid sensory and cognitive problems increases and can exacerbate the handicapping effects of hearing loss or make managing the hearing loss more challenging. It is well recognised that cognition declines with advancing age and has been shown to be associated with the ability of individuals with hearing loss to recognise speech sounds in the presence of fast and slow compression in hearing aids [20].

Conclusions

ARHL is a major public health problem that is expected to significantly increase with the ageing population. Currently, the management of ARHL is limited primarily to the fitting of devices with little support for the psychological and social consequences of hearing loss. Therefore, only approximately one-fourth of older adults with hearing loss currently seek hearing healthcare services. However, a more holistic understanding of the effects of hearing loss on the individuals, their significant others and the community might shift the focus of rehabilitation towards a more bio-psycho-social and environmental model which would focus on mitigating the handicapping effects of hearing loss through multiple strategies. These might include environmental, social and psychological supports, lessening the burden of hearing loss on the individuals and their significant others and increasing their social participation, ensuring that they remain active members of the community for longer. Certainly, while the cost of remediating hearing loss might appear to be substantial, economic analyses show that the loss of workplace productivity significantly exceeds this cost [21].

Acknowledgements

Thanks to Prof. Robert Cowan for his critical review of the manuscript. The author acknowledges the financial support of the HEARing CRC, established and supported under the funding from the Cooperative Research Centres Programme – Business Australia.

References

1 Scarinci N, Worrall L, Hickson L: The ICF and third-party disability: its application to spouses of older people with hearing impairment. Disabil Rehabil 2009;31:2088–2100.

2 Gates GA, Mills JH: Presbycusis. Lancet 2005;366:1111–1120.

3 Chia EM, Wang JJ, Rochtchina E, Cumming RR, Newall P, Mitchell P: Hearing impairment and health-related quality of life: the Blue Mountains Hearing Study. Ear Hear 2007;28:187–195.

4 Weinstein BE, Ventry IM: Hearing impairment and social isolation in the elderly. J Speech Hear Res 1982;25:593–599.

5 Cruickshanks KJ, Klein R, Klein BE, Wiley TL, Nondahl DM, Tweed TS: Cigarette smoking and hearing loss: the epidemiology of hearing loss study. JAMA 1998;279:1715–1719.

6 Steffens L, Venter K, O'Beirne GA, Kelly-Campbell R, Gibbs D, Bird P: The current state of ototoxicity monitoring in New Zealand. N Z Med J 2013;127:84–97.

7 World Health Organization: Hearing loss in persons 65 years and older. Mortality and Burden of Diseases and Prevention of Blindness and Deafness, 2012. http://www.who.int/pbd/deafness/news/GE_65years.pdf (accessed February 15, 2015).

8 Kelly HA, Weeks SA: Ear disease in three aboriginal communities in Western Australia. Med J Aust 1991; 154:240–245.

9 Dawes P, Fortnum H, Moore DR, Emsley R, Norman P, et al: Hearing in middle age: a population snapshot of 40-to 69-year olds in the United Kingdom. Ear Hear 2014;35:e44–e51.

10 Oyler AL: Untreated hearing loss in adults – a growing national epidemic. http://www.asha.org/Aud/Articles/Untreated-Hearing-Loss-in-Adults/ (accessed June 26, 2015).

11 McMahon CM, Kifley A, Rochtchina E, Newall P, Mitchell P: The contribution of family history to hearing loss in an older population. Ear Hear 2008;29: 578–584.

12 Karlsson K, Harris J, Svartengren M: Description and primary results from an audiometric study of male twins. Ear Hear 1997;18:114–120.

13 Christensen K, Frederiksen H, Hoffman HJ: Genetic and environmental influences on self-reported reduced hearing in the old and oldest old. J Am Geriatr Soc 2001;49:1512–1517.

14 Van Eyken E, Van Camp G, Van Laer L: The complexity of age-related hearing impairment: contributing environmental and genetic factors. Audiol Neurotol 2007;12:345–358.

15 Nomura K, Nakao M, Yano E: Hearing loss associated with smoking and occupational noise exposure in a Japanese metal working company. Int Arch Occup Environ Health 2005;78:178–184.

16 Daniel E: Noise and hearing loss: a review. J Sch Health 2007;77:225–231.

17 Basner M, Babisch W, Davis A, Brink M, Clark C, et al: Auditory and non-auditory effects of noise on health. Lancet 2014;383:1325–1332.

18 Gopinath B, Wang JJ, Schneider J, Burlutsky G, Snowdon J, McMahon CM, et al: Depressive symptoms in older adults with hearing impairments: The Blue Mountains Study. J Am Geriatr Soc 2009;57:1306–1308.

19 Ferrite S, Santana V: Joint effects of smoking, noise exposure and age on hearing loss. Occup Med 2005;55:48–53.

20 Lunner T: Cognitive function in relation to hearing aid use. Int J Audiol 2003; 42(suppl 1):S49–S58.

21 Access Economics: Listen Hear! The economic impact and cost of hearing loss in Australia. Access Economics, 2006. https://www.audiology.asn.au/public/1/files/Publications/Listen HearFinal.pdf.

22 Ruben RJ: Redefining the survival of the fittest: communication disorders in the 21st century. Laryngoscope 2000;110: 241–245.

23 Wallhagen MI: The stigma of hearing loss. Gerontologist 2010;50:66–75.

24 Knudsen LV, Öberg M, Nielsen C, Naylor G, Kramer SE: Factors influencing help seeking, hearing aid uptake, hearing aid use and satisfaction with hearing aids: a review of the literature. Trends Amplif 2010;14:127–154.

25 Gagné JP, Jennings MB, Southall K: The ICF: a classification system and conceptual framework ideal for audiological rehabilitation. SIG 7 Perspectives on Aural Rehabilitation and Its Instrumentation 2009;16:8–14.

26 Halfon N, Hochstein M: Life course health development: an integrated framework for developing health, policy, and research. Milbank Q 2002;80:433–479.

27 Morata TC: Young people: their noise and music exposures and the risk of hearing loss. Int J Audiol 2007;46:111–112.

28 Schweitzer VG: Ototoxicity of chemotherapeutic agents. Otolaryngol Clin North Am 1993;26:759–789.

29 World Health Organization: 1.1 Billion people at risk of hearing loss. 2015. http://www.who.int/mediacentre/news/releases/2015/ear-care/en/ (accessed May 19, 2015).

30 Nelson DI, Nelson RY, Concha-Barrientos M, Fingerhut M: The global burden of occupational noise-induced hearing loss. Am J Ind Med 2005;48:446–458.

31 Verbeek JH, Kateman E, Morata TC, Dreschler WA, Mischke C: Interventions to prevent occupational noise-induced hearing loss. Cochrane Database Syst Rev 2012;10:CD006396.

32 Smith PA, Davis A, Ferguson M, Lutman ME: The prevalence and type of social noise exposure in young adults in England. Noise Health 2000;2:41–56.

33 Kujawa SG, Liberman MC: Acceleration of age-related hearing loss by early noise exposure: evidence of a misspent youth. J Neurosci 2006;26:2115–2123.

34 Kujawa SG, Liberman MC: Adding insult to injury: cochlear nerve degeneration after 'temporary' noise-induced hearing loss. J Neurosci 2009;29:14077–14085.

35 Gourévitch B, Edeline JM, Occelli F, Eggermont JJ: Is the din really harmless? Long-term effects of non-traumatic noise on the adult auditory system. Nat Rev Neurosci 2014;15:483–491.

36 Gopinath B, Flood VM, McMahon CM, Burlutsky G, Brand-Miller J, Mitchell P: Dietary glycemic load is a predictor of age-related hearing loss in older adults. J Nutr 2010;140:2207–2212.

37 Gopinath B, Flood VM, Rochtchina E, McMahon CM, Mitchell P: Consumption of omega-3 fatty acids and fish and risk of age-related hearing loss. Am J Clin Nutr 2010;92:416–421.

38 Peel NM, McClure RJ, Bartlett HP: Behavioral determinants of healthy aging. Am J Prev Med 2005;28:298–304.

39 Rybak L, Ramkumar V: Ototoxicity. Kidney Int 2007;72:931–935.

40 Arslan E, Orzan E, Santarelli R: Global problem of drug-induced hearing loss. Ann N Y Acad Sci 1999;884:1–14.

41 Davis RR, Newlander JK, Ling XB, Cortopassi GA, Krieg EF, Erway LC: Genetic basis for susceptibility to noise-induced hearing loss in mice. Hear Res 2001;155: 82–90.

42 Pouryaghoub G, Mehrdad R, Mohammadi S: Interaction of smoking and occupational noise exposure on hearing loss: a cross-sectional study. BMC Public Health 2007;7:137.

43 Morata TC, Fiorini AC, Fischer FM, Colacioppo S, Wallingford KM, et al: Toluene-induced hearing loss among rotogravure printing workers. Scand J Work Environ Health 1997;23:289–298.

44 Frisina RD: Age-related hearing loss: ear and brain mechanisms. Ann N Y Acad Sci 2009;1170:708–717.

45 Gale CR, Martyn CN, Cooper C: Cognitive impairment and mortality in a cohort of elderly people. BMJ 1996;312: 608–611.

46 Dunn JE, Rudberg MA, Furner SE, Cassel CK: Mortality, disability, and falls in older persons: the role of underlying disease and disability. Am J Public Health 1992;82:395–400.

47 Albers MW, Gilmore GC, Kaye J, Murphy C, Wingfield A, et al: At the interface of sensory and motor dysfunctions and Alzheimer's disease. Alzheimers Dement 2015;11:70–98.

48 Lin FR, Albert M: Hearing loss and dementia – who is listening? Aging Ment Health 2014;18:671–673.

49 Lin FR, Metter EJ, O'Brien RJ, Resnick SM, Zonderman AB, Ferrucci L: Hearing loss and incident dementia. Arch Neurol 2011;68:214–220.

50 Uhlmann RF, Larson EB, Rees TS, Koepsell TD, Duckert LG: Relationship of hearing impairment to dementia and cognitive dysfunction in older adults. JAMA 1989;261:1916–1919.

51 Weinstein BE: Hearing loss and senile dementia in the institutionalized elderly. Clin Gerontologist 1986;4:3–15.

52 Viljanen A, Kaprio J, Pyykkö I, Sorri M, Pajala S, et al: Hearing as a predictor of falls and postural balance in older female twins. J Gerontol A Biol Sci Med Sci 2009;64:312–317.

53 Lin FR, Ferrucci L: Hearing loss and falls among older adults in the United States. Arch Intern Med 2012;172:369–371.

54 Marmot M: Social determinants of health inequalities. Lancet 2005;365: 1099–1104.

55 Chisolm TH, Johnson CE, Danhauer JL, Portz LJ, Abrams HB, et al: A systematic review of health-related quality of life and hearing aids: final report of the American Academy of Audiology Task Force on the Health-Related Quality of Life Benefits of Amplification in Adults. J Am Acad Audiol 2007;18:151–183.

56 Stephens SD, Callaghan DE, Hogan S, Meredith R, Rayment A, Davis AC: Hearing disability in people aged 50–65: effectiveness and acceptability of rehabilitative intervention. BMJ 1990;300: 508–511.

57 Davis A, Smith P, Ferguson M, Stephens D, Gianopoulos I: Acceptability, benefit and costs of early screening for hearing disability: a study of potential screening tests and models. Health Technol Assess 2007;11:1–294.

58 Hickson L, Meyer C, Lovelock K, Lampert M, Khan A: Factors associated with success with hearing aids in older adults. Int J Audiol 2014;53(suppl 1): S18–S27.

59 Meyer C, Hickson L: What factors influence help-seeking for hearing impairment and hearing aid adoption in older adults? Int J Audiol 2012;51:66–74.

60 Wänström G, Öberg M, Rydberg E, Lunner T, Laplante-Lévesque A, Andersson G: The psychological process from avoidance to acceptance in adults with acquired hearing impairment. Hearing, Balance and Communication 2014;12: 27–35.

61 Yorgason JB, Piercy FP, Piercy SK: Acquired hearing impairment in older couple relationships: an exploration of couple resilience processes. J Aging Stud 2007;21:215–228.

62 Schneider JM, Gopinath B, McMahon CM, Britt HC, Harrison CM, et al: Role of general practitioners in managing age-related hearing loss. Med J Aust 2010;192:20–23.

63 World Health Organization: Prevention of blindness and deafness. Grades of hearing impairment. 2015. http://www.who.int/pbd/deafness/hearing_impairment_grades/en/ (accessed January 29, 2015).

64 Hartley D, Rochtchina E, Newall P, Golding M, Mitchell P: Use of hearing aids and assistive listening devices in an older Australian population. J Am Acad Audiol 2010;21:642–653.

65 McCormack A, Fortnum H: Why do people fitted with hearing aids not wear them? Int J Audiol 2013;52:360–368.

66 Lowry KA, Vallejo AN, Studenski SA: Successful aging as a continuum of functional independence: lessons from physical disability models of aging. Aging Dis 2012;3:5–15.

67 Mikkola TM, Portegijs E, Rantakokko M, Gagné JP, Rantanen T, Viljanen A: Association of self-reported hearing difficulty to objective and perceived participation outside the home in older community-dwelling adults. J Aging Health 2015;27:103–122.

68 Genther DJ, Betz J, Pratt S, Kritchevsky SB, Martin KR, et al: Association of hearing impairment and mortality in older adults. J Gerontol A Biol Sci Med Sci 2015;70:85–90.

69 Schneider J, Gopinath B, Karpa MJ, McMahon CM, Rochtchina E, et al: Hearing loss impacts on the use of community and informal supports. Age Ageing 2010;39:458–464.

70 Rönnberg J, Lunner T, Zekveld A, Sörqvist P, Danielsson H, et al: The Ease of Language Understanding (ELU) model: theoretical, empirical, and clinical advances. Front Syst Neurosci 2013;7: 31.

Catherine M. McMahon
Department of Linguistics, Macquarie University
Balaclava Road, North Ryde
Sydney, NSW 2109 (Australia)
E-Mail cath.mcmahon@mq.edu.au

Vona B, Haaf T (eds): Genetics of Deafness. Monogr Hum Genet. Basel, Karger, 2016, vol 20, pp 19–29
(DOI: 10.1159/000444563)

Audiological Assessment and Management in the Era of Precision Medicine

Kevin J. Munro[a, b] · Valerie E. Newton[a] · David R. Moore[a, c]

[a]School of Psychological Sciences, The University of Manchester, and [b]Central Manchester University Hospitals NHS Foundation Trust, Manchester Academic Health Science Centre, Manchester, UK; [c]Cincinnati Children's Hospital Medical Center, Cincinnati, Ohio, USA

Abstract

Hearing loss (HL) is the most common sensory deficit in childhood. Infant hearing screening is becoming widespread, and effective early intervention leads to an improved outcome. Genetic causes account for 50–60% of HL in childhood. Genetic screening has the potential to identify individuals who pass the infant hearing screen but are at risk from late-onset/progressive HL. Otitis media (OM) is the most frequently diagnosed disease in childhood, but the majority of genes underlying OM susceptibility have yet to be identified. A number of genetic conditions, both syndromic and nonsyndromic, are associated with progressive HL, necessitating regular audiological assessment. At the other end of the lifespan, age-related hearing loss (ARHL) is a major disease burden. It is a complex disorder with environmental and genetic contributions. Despite a genetic contribution of 56–70%, genetic research into ARHL is relatively untapped. The effectiveness of adult hearing screening has not been established although simple internet-based speech-in-noise hearing tests could be readily implemented for large-scale screening. Hearing instruments are the primary treatment for permanent HL. It is likely that a precise genetic diagnosis, perhaps identifying the anatomical location of the HL, will increase personalisation of treatment and improve treatment outcome.

© 2016 S. Karger AG, Basel

The World Health Organisation (WHO) estimates that over 5% of the world's population, 360 million people (328 million adults and 32 million children), have a disabling hearing loss (HL) [1]. In 2004, the WHO estimated that HL was ranked 15th in terms of contribution to the global burden of disease: by 2030, this is expected to rise to 7th because of the growing global population and longer life expectancy [2]. Approximately one-third of people over 65 years of age are affected by disabling HL. In addition, permanent childhood hearing loss (PCHL; defined here as ≥40 dB HL averaged over 0.5, 1, 2, and 4 kHz), the most common sensory deficit, has a prevalence of at least 1–2/1,000 births [3]. Therefore, most individuals, or members of their family, will attend an audiology service at some point in their life.

Audiology is the 'science of hearing', but it is used in a health care setting to mean the study and assessment of hearing and balance problems and the treatment and prevention of disorders of these functions. In this review, we (1) provide an introduction to hearing and deafness, (2) discuss the increasing emphasis on personalisation and (3) indicate how genomic medicine is likely to impact on audiological assessment and management. A summary of common audiological procedures is provided in table 1. The interested reader is directed to the comprehensive textbooks on clinical audiology [4], paediatric audiology [5], and hearing instruments [6].

Screening for Hearing Loss in Children

PCHL is a potentially devastating long-term condition because of its negative impact on communication skills [7], learning and education [8], behaviour [9], mental health [10], employment opportunities [11], family dynamics [7], and quality of life [9]. Effective intervention by 6 months of age can significantly reduce the negative impact of PCHL on speech and language learning [12–15].

The WHO recommends that universal newborn hearing screening is adopted in all countries with appropriate rehabilitation services. Screening is a process of identifying apparently healthy individuals who may be at increased risk of a disease. Two different types of tests are used to screen for HL in babies: otoacoustic emissions and the auditory brainstem response (ABR). Both tests are reliable and can be used separately or together. An otoacoustic emission is a small amount of sound that is generated in the normal, healthy cochlea and can be measured with a small sensitive microphone in the ear canal [16]. The automated

ABR uses surface electrodes attached to the head to record neural activity evoked by sound.

In many countries, newborn hearing screening has become widespread, but it is almost non-existent in some regions of the world including sub-Saharan Africa and South-East Asia. Even when it is available, there is often great variation: some wealthy countries have fragmented and ineffective programmes, whilst a number of less-wealthy countries have very successful programmes. In countries that have hearing screening, and a high compliance with confirmatory testing, the age when intervention commences has dramatically reduced. For example, in England, the first country to have a universal newborn hearing screening programme, the typical age that a child with a significant congenital HL is first prescribed and fitted with hearing instruments has reduced from 300 days in 2006, when the phased introduction of newborn screening was completed, to 82 days in 2011 [17].

Despite the resounding success of some newborn hearing screening programmes at reducing the age of identification of HL, there are on-going challenges. For example, the diagnostic frequency-specific ABR is absent, or abnormal, in some clinical populations including those with auditory neuropathy spectrum disorder (ANSD). ANSD is a type of HL in which the outer hair cells within the cochlea are present and functioning, but sound is not faithfully transmitted to the auditory nerve (one branch of the vestibulocochlear nerve) and higher auditory pathways [18]. A growing number of genetic causes of ANSD are being identified [19] and could lead to the development of more effective and targeted treatments in babies born with this condition.

Newborn hearing screening does not identify individuals at risk from late-onset HL. As an adjunct to audiological screening, molecular genetic tests could provide the opportunity to identify infants at risk from late-onset and/or progressive HL. The potential benefits of screening for susceptibility to disease [20], particularly with reference

Table 1. Summary of common audiological procedures

Domain	Example of clinical test technique	Comment
Impairment	PTA	a technique for determining hearing threshold levels for pure tones by behavioural means; stimuli are applied monaurally via an earphone (termed air conduction), or vibrations may be applied via a vibrator to the skull (termed bone conduction)
	VRA	a technique for determining minimum response levels by behavioural means, usually a conditioned head turn, in the developmental age range 6–36 months
Disability	speech recognition test	usually involves repeating words or sentences presented in quiet or in a background noise; also used as outcome measure
	self-report questionnaire	can be used to determine the need for intervention or as an outcome measure
Handicap	self-report questionnaire	can be used to determine the need for intervention or as an outcome measure
Other	immittance audiometry	includes tympanometry and acoustic reflex thresholds and is primarily used to assess middle ear function, e.g. presence of middle ear effusion
	auditory evoked potentials	measurement of auditory function by means of externally recorded electrical potentials evoked by acoustic stimuli applied to the ear; techniques can be distinguished according to the site of origin, e.g. ABR, CAEP; most common application is to estimate hearing levels when behavioural assessment (e.g. PTA or VRA) is unreliable
	otoacoustic emissions	vibrational energy originating in the normal functioning cochlea which is observable as sound in the external ear canal; most common application is to screen for hearing loss, e.g. in newborn population
	probe-tube microphone measurements	used to measure sound level in the ear canal before and after the provision of amplification

ABR = Auditory brainstem response; CAEP = cortical auditory evoked potential; PTA = pure tone audiometry; VRA = visual reinforcement audiometry.

to hearing, have been summarised by others [21] but include (1) disease prevention, (2) improved treatment, (3) improved interpretation of the results of early intervention, and (4) the psychological benefits of understanding the true cause of the HL.

More than 50% of prelingual deafness is genetic, most often autosomal recessive and nonsyndromic. Approximately 50% of autosomal recessive nonsyndromic HL can be attributed to mutations in *GJB2*, the gene that encodes the gap junction protein Connexin 26.

Screening for Hearing Loss in Older Adults

At the other end of the lifespan continuum, age-related hearing loss (ARHL) is a complex disorder with contributions from both environmental and genetic factors [22]. Adults with ARHL commonly delay 10–15 years before seeking help [23]. Yet, we know that the consequences of uncorrected HL can be significant for the individuals and their communication partners. Difficulties experienced at home, work and in social interaction compromise participation, independence and quality of life [24]. Evidence shows that hearing instruments improve social functioning and quality of life, and long-term outcomes are better when they are obtained earlier [25].

A universal screening programme for detecting HL in older adults would identify those who would benefit from earlier intervention. Morris et al. [26] undertook a modelling exercise and demonstrated that adult hearing screening, using conventional pure tone audiometry (PTA), would be cost-effective; however, a randomised trial of adult hearing screening has yet to be published. With the rapid explosion of access to the internet, and the use of mobile technology, it is now possible to use a simple online speech-in-noise hearing test for reliable large-scale hearing screening [27]. Speech-in-noise hearing tests are easy to standardise, do not require a sound booth and are potentially better than PTA at identifying declining cognitive processing ability associated with reduced ability to hear speech [28].

Audiological Assessment

The most widely used assessment procedure for measuring HL is PTA [29]. The degree of HL can, and usually does, vary with frequency. The ability to hear speech is related to the degree of HL. The proportion of speech that is audible to a listener can be quantified using a procedure known as the speech intelligibility index [30].

Well-known examples of environmental risk (and protective) factors for ARHL include noise damage, ototoxic medications, alcohol, and tobacco [31]. However, genetic research into ARHL is a relatively new and untapped scientific area despite an estimated genetic contribution of 56–70% [32]. Currently, only around 8 genes have been reported to be associated with ARHL, and there are few published replications of these findings [33].

HL is generally divided into 2 categories: conductive and sensorineural. Conductive HL occurs when there is a problem in the outer or middle ear, which prevents sound being conducted to the cochlea in the inner ear. An example would be Treacher Collins syndrome, an autosomal dominant disorder, where the HL is the result of microtia and malformed ossicles. Sensorineural HL involves a problem with either the sensory transducer cells in the cochlea or, less commonly, the neural pathway to the brain. An example would be Pendred's syndrome, an autosomal recessive disorder, where the HL is due to a cochlear malformation. In some genetic conditions, such as branchio-oto-renal (BOR) syndrome and CHARGE syndrome (CHARGE stands for coloboma, heart defect, atresia choanae, retarded growth and development, genital abnormality, and ear abnormality), there is a combination of conductive and sensorineural HL, i.e. a mixed HL. A HL involving the auditory nerve (or the medial ascending auditory pathway) is described as a retrocochlear HL.

Conductive HL can often be corrected via surgery and, when acquired, is relatively common in childhood with more than 95% of children having an episode of otitis media (OM) with effusion before starting school [34]. Sensorineural HL is usually permanent. Therefore, it is important to distinguish between the 2 categories. This is most commonly achieved by comparing air conduction and bone conduction hearing threshold levels. Disorders of any part of the auditory pathway will affect the air conduction threshold but disorders of the conducting mechanism will have much less effect on bone conduction measurements since these generally bypass the outer and middle ear.

The dynamic range between the threshold of hearing and loudness discomfort level is around 80–100 dB in normal hearing listeners. Unlike individuals with a pure conductive HL, listeners having a sensory HL will have raised hearing thresholds but their loudness discomfort levels will be essentially similar to normal hearing listeners. These individuals have a reduced dynamic range and an abnormal rate of loudness growth: this is known as loudness recruitment, i.e. an abnormally disproportionate increase in loudness for a small increase in intensity. This has implications for the design of hearing instruments. While a hearing instrument with multichannel compression can compensate by providing more amplification for soft sounds, relative to loud sounds, they are not able to compensate for the loss of supra-threshold abilities such as impaired frequency resolution (the ability to distinguish between different frequency components that occur simultaneously). This means that hearing in background noise remains problematic for most people with a HL, despite the ubiquitous use of directional microphone technology and noise reduction algorithms in modern digital hearing instruments.

A number of genetic conditions are associated with progressive HL, necessitating regular assessment. These include nonsyndromic HL as well as syndromes, e.g. Pendred's syndrome, neurofibromatosis type 2, BOR syndrome, Usher syndrome type 3, and Alport syndrome.

Pendred's syndrome is associated with an enlarged vestibular aqueduct. This abnormality can be found alone or in conjunction with other syndromes such as BOR and CHARGE syndrome. This radiological abnormality is associated with fluctuation and deterioration in hearing. Where an enlarged vestibular aqueduct is present, mild head trauma is sufficient to precipitate a reduction in hearing, and the progression can be sudden and severe [35]. In individuals with Alport's syndrome, a sensorineural HL usually appears in the first decade. A further example is asymptomatic neurofibromatosis type 2. In most cases, progressive sensorineural HL occurs in the second decade, but in a few cases, it can occur in the first decade [36].

There are a number of pharmacological products that are ototoxic including some antibiotics (e.g. aminoglycosides), loop diuretics and chemotherapeutic agents (e.g. including cisplatin and carboplatin). Approximately 1/500 individuals carry a mitochondrial mutation, which is associated with profound HL caused by gentamicin.

Other Audiological Assessment Techniques

Between a developmental age of 6 months and 3 years, the hearing assessment of choice is visual reinforcement audiometry. This involves pairing a head-turn response to a sound with an interesting visual reward such as a flashing light or an animated toy animal. Once this classical conditioning has been established, operant conditioning then takes place where a visual reward is presented after an appropriate sound-elicited head turn. This technique is used to determine the minimum response level that will elicit a head turn.

Prior to 6 months of age, it is not possible to obtain reliable information using current behavioural methods of hearing assessment [37]. Although the observations of parents and professionals are important [38], the range of observable behaviour in infants is limited [39]. Event-related potentials can be used to estimate hearing sensitivity. The method of choice in infants is the frequency-specific ABR because this can be obtained during sleep or under sedation. A typical clinical protocol would be to commence at a high sound level and reduce in level until the evoked response can no longer be detected. The presence of a response is usually based on subjective interpretation of the waveform by the tester. An alternative technique that is gaining popularity is the auditory steady state response, which has the benefit that response presence is based on objective, online, statistical analysis. Auditory evoked potentials, primarily the obligatory cortical auditory evoked potential, can also be used to estimate hearing sensitivity in adults who are unable or unwilling to provide reliable information via PTA.

Historically, auditory evoked potentials have had a valuable diagnostic role, especially when identifying tumours associated with the auditory nerve, but tumour identification is now largely achieved using advanced diagnostic imaging techniques. However, event-related potentials continue to be used for research purposes and may, for example, have a diagnostic role in the detection of neural degeneration and suprathreshold deficits in individuals with normal hearing thresholds who complain of aberrant auditory perceptions such as tinnitus and hyperacusis [40].

A commonly used procedure that provides information about the condition of the eardrum and the middle ear is known as tympanometry. Although this can also be applied in adults, it is particularly useful in children because of the high incidence of OM. The procedure works on the principle that some sound entering the ear canal is reflected back from the eardrum, and this can be measured with a sensitive microphone. Stiffening the eardrum by changing the pressure of the air trapped in the ear canal should result in more sound being reflected by the eardrum. However, if there is fluid in the middle ear, then the stiffness of the eardrum will be unaffected by changing the air pressure in the ear canal.

Well-known examples of environmental risk factors for OM include day care attendance, cigarette smoke exposure and bottle feeding. Daly et al. [41] were the first to demonstrate that parents and siblings of affected children with OM had a greater than expected rate of OM based on population rates. Exploration of genetic influences in OM is in its early stages and the majority of genes underlying this susceptibility are, as yet, unidentified. Mouse models of OM are an important component of current approaches to understand the complex genetic susceptibility to OM in humans [42]. In order to determine common variants contributing to OM susceptibility, Allen et al. [43] performed the first genome-wide association study on OM and identified a novel susceptibility locus on chromosome 2.

Audiological Management

Acoustic hearing instruments, provided in the context of patient-centred, minimally disruptive medicine, are the primary treatment for permanent HL. The hearing instrument prescription and fitting protocol has 3 primary objectives: (1) to restore the audibility of soft sounds, (2) to provide improved intelligibility of speech for low and medium input sound levels, and (3) to ensure that intense sounds are not amplified to an uncomfortably loud level.

The hearing instrument fitting process commences with an assessment of (1) impairment, (2) hearing ability in different listening situations, (3) the ability to participate in activities that require good hearing, and (4) motivation and expectations. In the clinical setting, hearing problems are most frequently assessed using PTA and supplemented, in some countries, with speech recognition measures. The remaining components of the assessment often involve the use of standardised self-report questionnaires.

The selection of appropriate amplification will include decisions about the fitting arrangement (e.g. bilateral vs. unilateral), style (e.g. behind-the-ear versus in-the-ear), coupling (e.g. standard earmould or an 'open' fitting), specific features (e.g. the need for a volume control), and amplification characteristics of the device. The detection of environmental sounds, appreciation of music and spatial hearing are also important considerations. The main goal, however, of providing amplification is to improve functional auditory capacity and restore good communication skills. The starting point for achieving this goal is to establish appropriate amplification characteristics for the individual.

Since the degree and configuration of HL vary from one person to the next, it is not appropriate to provide the same amplification characteristics to all individuals with a HL. Personalised amplification characteristics are most commonly selected using pure tone hearing thresholds. In general, there are few established amplification prescription rationales that rely on supra-threshold data. However, the discovery of 'hidden HL', a supra-threshold deficit resulting from ageing or noise exposure, but having no impact on hearing thresholds [44], emphasises the need for further research on supra-threshold psychometric and physiological measures.

The literature on amplification prescription approaches is as confusing as it is voluminous. There are many different prescription rationales, with significant variations in amplification target values for the same HL, and little evidence that one validated method results in greater benefit to the individual than another. Many hearing instrument manufacturers have also developed their own proprietary prescription fitting algorithm. In general, proprietary prescription methods are geared toward 'first acceptance' rather than restoring audibility and intelligibility. Current hearing instrument fitting guidelines recommend the use of generic validated prescription methods. Since many individuals will undergo changes in their hearing thresholds over time, this will necessitate regular assessments and, where necessary, a change in the amplification prescription targets.

In the field of healthcare, there is increasing emphasis on personalisation of treatment. This is done with the intention of accounting for individual variations and improving treatment outcomes. Hearing instrument prescriptions are based on the audiometric profile of the individual, so they already contain an element of personalisation. However, recent prescription methods take this personalisation a step further by accounting for additional factors such as listening experience, gender, language, and listening environment. For example, the amplification prescription for a congenital and an acquired HL is different. The reason for this is that adult hearing instrument users with an acquired HL, especially new users, prefer aided listening levels below those of children with a HL [45]. Thus, the prescription formula is now based on 'preference' in addition to audibility and loudness.

Adjusting a hearing instrument to match an amplification prescription target is most commonly verified using a probe-microphone system, a procedure that involves placing a small microphone in the patient's ear canal. Probe-microphone measurements require the passive cooperation of the individual, and this can be a challenge with infants and young children. For this reason, an alternative method of prescription verification is required for young children. One approach is to simulate the real ear by measuring hearing instrument performance in a standard test cavity, known as a 2-cc coupler, and then adding a correction to account for the difference between the ear and the standard coupler [46]. Several studies have demonstrated the validity of using this simulated real ear approach to verify the hearing instrument prescription [47].

Numerous studies have revealed the extent to which the acoustic properties of the ear canal change during the first few years of life. As a child grows, the ear canal increases in volume and the difference between the real ear and the standard coupler, becomes smaller. However, as with all anthropometric measurements, there is significant interpersonal variability [48]. For this reason, it is advisable to measure the correction factor for each individual, although the similarity between the right and left ear means that it may only be necessary to measure the correction factor in one ear of the child [49].

There are a number of hearing instrument features (e.g. frequency lowering, directional microphone, digital noise reduction, and automatic feedback reduction) that the audiologist may wish to verify. Whilst precise characterisation of these features may not be possible in the clinical setting, it is possible to use real-ear probe-microphone measurements to perform a few simple measurements that indicate if the features are broadly working as expected.

Alternative Auditory Prostheses

Individuals with a profound HL obtain little benefit from a conventional acoustic hearing instrument. However, direct electrical stimulation can be provided to the auditory nerve using a device known as a cochlear implant (CI). CIs have proved to be extremely successful and are arguably the most effective neural prostheses ever developed. Implantation is applicable even when there is a Mondini malformation of the cochlea, as in several genetic conditions, e.g. Pendred's syndrome and CHARGE syndrome. It has been suggested that this is successful because most of the spiral ganglion cells are in the basal turn of the cochlea, and so sufficient stimulation can be provided by the CI [50].

In general, the outcome of implantation is extremely variable, and attempts are being made to understand differences between individuals. It is possible that a precise genetic diagnosis may help understand these differences. Because the CI bypasses the membranous labyrinth within the cochlea but relies on the spiral ganglion for functionality, CI performance may be influenced, at

least in part, by the anatomical location of the HL. This is supported by preliminary data suggesting that genes preferentially expressed in the spiral ganglion are indicative of poor CI performance, while mutations in genes expressed in the membranous labyrinth are indicative of a good outcome [51].

There are a number of other technologies that are used by a relatively small proportion of people with HL. Individuals with a unilateral HL may benefit from placing a microphone on the ear that is deaf and routing the signal to the normal hearing ear. This type of device is known as a CROS (contralateral routing of sound) aid, and it allows the individual to detect sounds from the deaf side. More recently, unilateral HL has been treated with a CI, and this is reported to improve sound localisation and speech recognition-in-noise [52], and reduce tinnitus [53].

Bone conduction instruments are suitable for individuals who have a large conductive HL or are unable to wear a conventional acoustic hearing instrument for medical or anatomical reasons. These devices bypass the outer and middle ear by stimulating the cochlea via mechanical vibration of the skull. There is also a novel intra-oral bone conduction device [54]. A popular type of bone conduction hearing instrument is the bone-anchored aid in which the vibrations are transmitted via an embedded titanium screw.

A promising new development is the 'Earlens Photonic' system (www.earlenscorp.com). This has a novel form of sound delivery with power and audio signal transmitted via light. The potential benefit of this technology is superior sound quality due to a smooth, wideband frequency response and low distortion.

Measuring Outcome

Traditional measures of outcome and benefit from hearing instruments involve the recognition of speech (e.g. single words or sentences) presented in the quiet or against a background of noise. These are a direct and objective way to measure the benefit provided by a hearing instrument and, in recent times, have relied on computer-based presentation and scoring. There is some controversy regarding the rate and extent of perceptual learning that occurs when sounds are re-reintroduced after a period of deprivation [55]. Current thinking is that speech recognition measures should be relatively stable from around 4–6 weeks after hearing instrument prescription and fitting.

Individuals with HL often describe listening as being effortful and taxing. A reliable measure of this listening effort, and the resulting fatigue, would be of considerable value. By tapping into a consequence of HL not otherwise captured by speech recognition tests, measures of listening effort and fatigue may provide a more comprehensive evaluation of hearing disability [56].

A major difficulty when measuring hearing instrument benefit in clinical trials, and in the clinical setting, is the inability to use blinding. Dawes et al. [57] have demonstrated that placebo effects are a source of bias in non-blinded hearing instrument trials. The influence of bias in the clinical setting from the expectations of the patient and/or the audiologist has received little attention to date.

In recent times, there has been a strong emphasis on assessment of benefit using validated self-report questionnaires. Health policy makers prefer generic measures of health-related quality of life that allow them to make comparisons across health conditions. However, the relative rankings of different diseases, and the change in utility associated with different interventions, differ according to the measure chosen [58]. For example, the Health Utilities Index mark 3 [59] is more sensitive to HL than the Medical Outcomes Study Short Form 36 (SF36) [60] because it includes questions specific to hearing.

The most common outcome measures used to guide personalised management strategies in au-diology are disease-specific self-report inventories. A vast array of these measures is available to assess aspects of outcome, including usage, benefit, residual difficulties, and satisfaction. It is usual to wait 3–4 months after hearing instrument prescription and fitting before measuring benefit since this is usually sufficient for the patient to become familiar with the device but long enough to reduce the chances of cognitive bias from the 'halo effect', a tendency to feel more positive about a recently acquired device.

In very recent times, it has become possible to measure device usage objectively because modern digital hearing instruments have the capacity to store information about the usage and daily pattern of use. This data-logging feature extends to classifying the listening environment and storing information about the use of the hearing instrument in each environment. Thus, big data sets are now available to optimise and personalise intervention.

Final Comments

HL is a major disease burden. It is the most common sensory deficit in childhood and in the elderly. Examples of genetic developments that could improve audiological assessment and management include: (1) molecular genetic testing to identify infants at high risk from progressive or late-onset HL who will not be identified by the infant hearing screen, (2) a better understanding of the genetic basis for susceptibility to OM, the most frequently diagnosed disease in childhood, (3) introduction of point of care tests for pharmacological-related ototoxicity, (4) identification of susceptibility genes in ARHL in order to provide possible targets for treatment and/or prevention of ARHL, and (5) a precise genetic diagnosis in permanent HL so that treatment can be personalised and variability in treatment outcome reduced.

References

1 World Health Organisation: Deafness and hearing loss. Fact sheet 300, updated March 2015. http://www.who.int/mediacentre/factsheets/fs300/en/.

2 World Health Organisation: Global Burden of Disease: 2004 update. Geneva, World Health Organisation, 2008. http://www.who.int/healthinfo/global_burden_disease/GBD_report_2004update_full.pdf.

3 Fortnum HM, Summerfield AQ, Marshall DH, Davis AC, Bamford JM: Prevalence of childhood hearing impairment in the United Kingdom and implications for universal neonatal hearing screening: questionnaire based ascertainment study. BMJ 2001;323:536–540.

4 Katz J, Chasin M, English K, Hood LJ, Tillery KL: Handbook of Clinical Audiology, ed 7. London, Wolters Kluwer, 2014.

5 Seewald RC, Tharpe AM: Comprehensive Handbook of Paediatric Audiology. San Diego, Plural Publishing, 2010.

6 Dillon H: Hearing Aids, ed 2. Stuttgart, Thieme, 2012.

7 Gregory S: Deaf Children and Their Families. Cambridge, Cambridge University Press, 1995.

8 Stacey PC, Fortnum HM, Barton GR, Summerfield AQ: Hearing-impaired children in the United Kingdom, I: auditory performance, communication skills, educational achievements, quality of life, and cochlear implantation. Ear Hear 2006;27:161–186.

9 Hind S, Davis A: Outcomes for children with permanent hearing impairment, in Seewald RC (ed): A Sound Foundation through Early Amplification. Proceedings of an International Conference. Staefa, Phonak AG, 2000, pp 199–212.

10 Hindley PA, Hill PD, McGuigan S, Kitson N: Psychiatric disorder in deaf and hearing impaired children and young people: a prevalence study. J Child Psychol Psychiatry 1994;35:917–934.

11 Punch R, Creed PA, Hyde M: Predicting career development in hard-of-hearing adolescents in Australia. J Deaf Stud Deaf Educ 2005;10:146–160.

12 Yoshinago-Itano C, Sedey AL, Coulter DK, Mehl A: Language of early- and later-identified children with hearing loss. Paediatrics 1998;102:1161–1171.

13 Moeller MP, Hoover B, Putman C, Arbataitis K, Bohnenkamp G, et al: Vocalizations of infants with hearing loss compared to infants with normal hearing: Part I – Phonetic development. Ear Hear 2007;28:605–627.

14 Moeller MP, Hoover B, Putman C, Arbataitis K, Bohnenkamp G, et al: Vocalizations of infants with hearing loss compared to infants with normal hearing: Part II – Transition to words. Ear Hear 2007;28:628–642.

15 Ching TYC, Dillon H, Hou S, Zhang V, Day J, et al: A randomized controlled comparison of NAL and DSL prescriptions for young children: hearing-aid characteristics and performance outcomes at three years of age. Int J Audiol 2013;52(suppl 2):S17–S28.

16 Kemp DT: Stimulated acoustic emissions from within the human auditory system. J Acoust Soc Am 1978;64:1386–1391.

17 Wood SA, Sutton GJ, Davis AC: Performance and characteristics of the newborn hearing screening programme in England: the first seven years. Inter J Audiol 2015;54:353–358.

18 Roush P, Frymark T, Venediktov R, Wang B: Audiologic management of auditory neuropathy spectrum disorder in children: a systematic review of the literature. Am J Audiol 2011;20:159–170.

19 Manchaiah VK, Zhao F, Danesh AA, Duprey R: The genetic basis of auditory neuropathy spectrum disorder (ANSD). Int J Pediatr Otorhinolaryngol 2011;75:151–158.

20 Khoury MJ, McCabe LL, McCabe ERB: Population screening in the age of genomic medicine. N Engl J Med 2003;348:50–58.

21 Schimmenti LA, Martinez A, Fox M, Crandall B, Shapiro N, et al: Genetic testing as part of the early hearing detection and intervention (EHDI) process. Genet Med 2004;6:521–525.

22 Van Eyken E, Van Camp G, Van Lear L: The complexity of age-related hearing impairment: contributing environmental and genetic factors. Audiol Neurotol 2007;12:345–358.

23 Davis A, Smith P, Ferguson M, Stephens D, Gianopoulos I: Acceptability, benefit and costs of early screening for hearing disability: a study of potential screening tests and models. Health Technol Assess 2007;11:1–294.

24 Arlinger S: Negative consequences of uncorrected hearing loss – a review. Int J Audiol 2003;42(suppl 2):S217–S220.

25 Chisholm T, Johnson C, Danhauer JA, Portz LJ, Abrams HB, et al: A systematic review of health-related quality of life and hearing aids: final report of the American Academy of Audiology Task Force on health-related quality of life benefits of amplification in adults. J Am Acad Audiol 2007;18:151–183.

26 Morris AE, Lutman ME, Cook AJ, Turner D: An economic evaluation of screening 60- to 70-year-old adults for hearing loss. J Public Health 2013;35:139–146.

27 Dawes P, Fortnum H, Moore DR, Emsley R, Norman P, et al: Hearing in middle age: a population snapshot of 40- to 69-year olds in the United Kingdom. Ear Hear 2014;35:e44–e51.

28 Moore DR, Edmondson-Jones M, Dawes P, Fortnum H, McCormack A, et al: Relations between speech-in-noise threshold, hearing loss and cognition from 40–69 years of age. PLoS One 2014;9:e107720.

29 Johnson EW: Tuning forks to audiometers and back again. Laryngoscope 1970;80:49–68.

30 American National Standards Institute: ANSI S3.5. American national standard methods for the calculation of the speech intelligibility index. New York, American National Standards Institute, 1997.

31 Dawes P, Cruickshanks KJ, Moore DR, Edmondson-Jones M, McCormack A, et al: Cigarette smoking, passive smoking, alcohol consumption, and hearing loss. J Assoc Res Otolaryngol 2014;15:663–674.

32 Wolber LE, Steves CJ, Spector TD, Williams FMK: Hearing ability with age in Northern European women: a new web-based approach to genetic studies. PLoS One 2012;7:e35500.

33 Dawes P, Platt H, Horan M, Ollier W, Munro KJ, et al: No association between apolipoprotein E or N-acetyltransferase 2 gene polymorphisms and age-related hearing loss. Laryngoscope 2015;125:e33–e38.

34 Halliday LF, Moore DR: Auditory basis of language and learning disorders; in Plack CJ (ed): The Oxford Handbook of Auditory Science: Hearing. Oxford, Oxford University Press, 2010, pp 349–374.

35 Parker M, Bitner-Glindzicz M: Genetic investigations in childhood deafness. Arch Dis Child 2015;100:271–278.

36 Evans DJR, Birch JM, Ramsden RT: Paediatric presentation of type 2 neurofibromatosis. Arch Dis Child 1999;81: 496–499.

37 Widen J: Adding objectivity to infant behavioral audiometry. Ear Hear 1993; 14:49–57.

38 Bagatto MP, Moodie ST, Malandrino AC, Richert FM, Clench DA, Scollie SD: The University of Western Ontario Pediatric Audiological Monitoring Protocol (UWO PedAMP). Trends Amplif 2011;15:57–76.

39 Bess FH, Humes LE: Audiology: the Fundamentals, ed 3. Philadelphia, Lippincott Williams & Wilkins, 2003.

40 Schaette R, McAlpine D: Tinnitus with a normal audiogram: physiological evidence for hidden hearing loss and computational model. J Neurosci 2011;31: 13452–13457.

41 Daly KA, Rich SS, Levine S, Margolis RH, Le CT, et al: The family study of otitis media: design and disease and risk factor profiles. Genet Epidemiol 1996; 13:451–468.

42 Rye MS, Bhutta MF, Cheeseman MT, Burgner D, Blackwell JM, et al: Unraveling the genetics of otitis media: from mouse to human and back again. Mamm Genome 2011;22:66–82.

43 Allen EK, Chen WM, Weeks DE, Chen F, Hou X, et al: A genome-wide association study of chronic otitis media with effusion and recurrent otitis media identifies a novel susceptibility locus on chromosome 2. J Assoc Res Otolaryngol 2013;14:791–800.

44 Plack CJ, Barker D, Prendergast G: Perceptual consequences of 'hidden' hearing loss. Trends Hear 2014;18: 2331216514550621.

45 Scollie SD, Seewald R, Cornelisse L, Moodie S, Bagatto M, et al: The Desired Sensation Level multistage input/output algorithm. Trends Amplif 2005;9:159–197.

46 Moodie KS, Seewald RC, Sinclair ST: Procedure for predicting real-ear hearing aid performance in young children. Am J Audiol 1994;3:23–31.

47 Munro KJ, Hatton N: Customized acoustic transform functions and their accuracy at predicting real-ear hearing aid performance. Ear Hear 2000;1:59–69.

48 Bagatto M, Scollie SD, Seewald RC, Moodie KS, Hoover BM: Real-ear-to-coupler difference predictions as a function of age for two coupling procedures. J Am Acad Audiol 2002;13:407–415.

49 Munro KJ, Howlin EM: Comparison of real-ear to coupler difference values in the right and left ear of hearing aid users. Ear Hear 2010;31:146–150.

50 Sennaroglu L: Cochlear implantation in inner ear malformations – a review article. Cochlear Implants Int 2010;11: 4–41.

51 Eppsteiner RW, Shearer AE, Hildebrand MS, Deluca AP, Ji H, et al: Prediction of cochlear implant performance by genetic mutation: the spiral ganglion hypothesis. Hear Res 2012;292:51–58.

52 Vermeire K, Van de Heyning P: Binaural hearing after cochlear implantation in subjects with unilateral sensorineural deafness and tinnitus. Audiol Neurotol 2009;14:163–171.

53 Arts R, George E, Stokroos R, Vermeire K: Review: cochlear implants as a treatment of tinnitus in single-sided deafness. Curr Opin Otolaryngol Head Neck Surg 2012;20:398–403.

54 Popelka GR, Derebery J, Blevins NH, Murray M, Moore BCJ, et al: Preliminary evaluation of a novel bone-conduction device for single-sided deafness. Otol Neurotol 2010;31:492–497.

55 Munro KJ: Reorganisation of the adult auditory system: perceptual and physiological evidence from monaural fitting of hearing aids. Trends Amplif 2008;12: 254–271.

56 McGarrigle R, Munro KJ, Dawes P, Stewart AJ, Moore DR, et al: Listening effort and fatigue: what exactly are we measuring? A British Society of Audiology Cognition in Hearing Special Interest Group 'white paper'. Int J Audiol 2014;53:433–445.

57 Dawes P, Hopkins R, Munro KJ: Placebo effects in hearing-aid trials are reliable. Int J Audiol 2013;52:472–477.

58 Barton GR, Bankart J, Davis AC, Summerfield QA: Comparing utility scores before and after hearing-aid provision: results according to the EQ-5D, HUI3 and SF-6D. Appl Health Econ Health Policy 2004;3:103–105.

59 Feeny D, Furlong W, Torrance GW, Goldsmith CH, Zhu Z, et al: Multi-attribute and single-attribute utility functions for the health utilities index mark 3 system. Med Care 2002;40:113–128.

60 Ware JE, Sherbourne CD: The MOS 36-item short-form health survey (SF-36). I. Conceptual framework and item selection. Med Care 1992;30:473–483.

Kevin J. Munro
School of Psychological Sciences, The University of Manchester
Ellen Wilkinson Building, Room A3.11
Oxford Road, Manchester M13 9PL (UK)
E-Mail kevin.j.munro@manchester.ac.uk

Vona B, Haaf T (eds): Genetics of Deafness. Monogr Hum Genet. Basel, Karger, 2016, vol 20, pp 30–39
(DOI: 10.1159/000444598)

Next-Generation Newborn Hearing Screening

Jun Shen · Cynthia C. Morton

Harvard Medical School Center for Hereditary Deafness, Brigham and Women's Hospital, Harvard Medical School, Boston, Mass., USA

Abstract

Hearing loss is the most common sensory deficit in humans. Untreated hearing loss will affect speech and language development and lead to impaired cognitive and social skills. Early detection and intervention have proven critical to successful rehabilitation and help individuals with hearing loss to reach their full potential. Since the adoption of universal newborn hearing screening in the United States and other parts of the world, many infants with congenital hearing loss have received a diagnosis shortly after birth and benefited from early intervention programs by 6 months of age, the critical period for language acquisition. However, traditional screening methods have their limitations, including high false positive and false negative rates, difficulty to distinguish transient versus permanent hearing loss, inability to prevent hearing loss presymptomatically, and no etiological explanations. New advances in next-generation sequencing and computing technologies have enabled rapid discoveries of genetic causes of hearing loss. Targeted therapeutic strategies hold the promise for precision medicine to treat hearing loss. Next-generation newborn hearing screening will incorporate comprehensive genomic analyses, which is expected to offer improved sensitivity, specificity, precise etiology, and an earlier window of opportunity for treatment to patients, and to reduce healthcare costs and disparities in society.   © 2016 S. Karger AG, Basel

Causes of Congenital Hearing Loss

Hearing loss may be acquired or inherited. Infection, ototoxic drugs, trauma, and noise exposure are known environmental risk factors for hearing loss. In utero infection due to cytomegalovirus (CMV) [1–3], toxoplasmosis [4–6], herpes [7], rubella [8], syphilis [9], etc. and childhood meningitis are associated with congenital hearing loss, with CMV infection being the most common [10]. Hospitalization in the neonatal intensive care unit (NICU) increases the risk for hearing loss by 10-fold [11], which could be due to the medical condition that necessitates being in the NICU, procedures performed in the NICU (e.g. extracorporeal membrane oxygenation [12, 13]), administration of ototoxic drugs during NICU stay (e.g. aminoglycosides), and noise exposure in the NICU. Ototoxic drugs including aminoglycoside antibiotics (e.g. gentamicin), loop diuretics (e.g. furosemide), platinum-based chemotherapy agents (e.g. cisplatin), and some nonsteroidal anti-inflammatory drugs have been shown to cause sensorineural hearing loss. It is well known that certain genetic variants in the mitochondrial 12S ribosomal RNA gene predispose carriers of these variants to aminoglycoside ototoxicity [14]. A recent study has linked common variants in *ACYP2* and susceptibility to cisplatin-induced hearing loss [15]. These exemplify that genetic factors affect an individual's susceptibility to certain environmental insults, hinting at the presence of more risk genes.

The majority of congenital hearing loss cases are hereditary. It can present as syndromic (accompanied by pathology in other organ systems), or nonsyndromic (where deafness is the only apparent anomaly). Hearing loss is a component in over 600 known syndromes [16]. An estimated 80% of cases of nonsyndromic hearing loss in developed countries are due to genetic factors [17]. Many syndromic forms of hearing loss may present as nonsyndromic in a newborn, because symptoms involving other organ systems may not have manifested yet.

The large number of currently known genes and implicated loci reflect unparalleled genetic heterogeneity in the etiology of hearing loss. To date, >150 nonsyndromic hearing loss loci (59 autosomal dominant, 90 autosomal recessive, 6 X-linked, and 1 Y-linked) have been reported, but the causative genes have been discovered in only 87 (33 dominant, 57 recessive, and 4 X-linked, including 7 involved in both dominant and recessive inheritance patterns) [18–20]. Pathogenic variants in *GJB2* (encoding connexin 26) account for ~25% of hereditary hearing loss [21]. Given the complexity of the hearing organ, many more genetic causes of hearing loss are being discovered on an ongoing basis at a rapid pace. Although hearing loss has been reported in >600 syndromes, <150 genes have been identified with evidence for causality. Hence, many more hearing loss genes await discovery.

Importance of Newborn Hearing Screening

Hearing loss is the most common sensory deficit in humans. One in 500 babies is born with hearing loss [22] and the prevalence increases to 1 in 100 by school age [23, 24]. Helen Keller's remark, 'Blindness separates people from things; deafness separates people from people,' hits the nail on the head. Hearing is essential to language and social development. Unattended hearing loss in young children results in compromised cognitive abilities, creates a communication barrier, and leads to social isolation, decreased employment opportunities and economic status, and subpar quality of life. Even when the hearing loss cannot be cured, accurate diagnosis will allow a family to cope with the condition in a timely manner. For example, introduction of sign language and eligibility to receive early intervention services can start as soon as hearing loss is identified. Early intervention has proven effective to mitigate some of the adverse consequences of hearing loss. However, it depends upon early detection of hearing loss – ideally prior to the onset of a significant loss.

Knowing the precise genetic etiology of hearing loss directly impacts patient care in many ways. First, accurate genetic diagnosis helps guide the best course of possible intervention and treatment. Genetic information can predict prognosis and determine the best management and rehabilitation option. Hearing aids, cochlear implants, auditory brainstem implants, and sign language are currently available habilitations to manage hearing loss [25]. The best choice and outcome of the management approach depends upon the underlying pathophysiological deficits and the timing of intervention [26–28]. As more genotype/phenotype correlations are being catalogued, genetic diagnosis will provide precise diagnoses and prognosis to dictate appropriate interventions. For example, an increasing number of studies are evaluating the effectiveness of cochlear implants based on the affected gene and its function, and localization in the cochlea and along the entire auditory processing pathway [16].

Second, genetic diagnosis of hearing loss in presymptomatic patients can allow careful monitoring to catch the optimal therapeutic window for hearing loss or other associated syndromic complications as well as to minimize environmental insults that can worsen disease. When a newborn presents with hearing loss, it may not be evident that other (occult) anomalies (e.g. not readily visible or in presymptomatic organ systems) may also be present. Even if other anomalies are observed, the exact syndrome and the possible presence of additional pathology may not be readily recognized. In these cases, management and care of the patient can fall short of all possible ramifications of the disorder. Jervell and Lange-Nielsen syndrome and sinoatrial node dysfunction and deafness involve abnormalities in hearing and cardiac function. Heart malfunction in affected individuals may go undetected, until it manifests as sudden death. Hence, accurate genetic diagnosis can translate into crucial information that would reveal the need for careful examination and work-up of other organ systems, and a much different course of management than with the clinical diagnosis of hearing loss alone.

Third, definitive genetic test results can, in many cases, eliminate the need for other expensive, uncomfortable or even harmful diagnostic tests that, for instance, require the use of sedatives or exposure to radiation in young children. This information would be valuable not only to the patient in terms of avoiding unnecessary, invasive, and costly procedures, but also to the overall state and cost of medical care. Genetic testing could facilitate limiting radiation exposure and sedation in infants due to computed tomography and magnetic resonance imaging studies to minimal necessities.

Fourth, genetic information can inform recurrence risks to family members and future children. The information is particularly useful in cases where the hearing loss or associated syndromic features are not readily detectable during early childhood. A couple may make a different reproductive decision depending on the health status of their current child. Next-generation newborn hearing screening offers them the opportunity to make a choice that would not have been possible until the current child is diagnosed with the existing standard of care.

Furthermore, identification of not only the gene, but also the exact variant, is often indicative of a particular nature, severity, course of disease, and mode of inheritance, which in turn dictates optimal strategies for management. New gene therapy strategies have recently become available [29–32]. Identification of the precise causal variant is required for those highly specific strategies to work. Recent successful targeted therapeutic correction of other human diseases [33, 34] or animal models with hearing loss [29–31, 35–37] by stem cells, antisense oligonucleotides, interference RNA or gene transfer has demonstrated the potential of targeted gene therapy to restore inner ear function. In summary, early diagnosis of a genetic etiology is crucial to successful management of hearing loss, and identification of the causative genetic variants will reveal the targets for effective precision medicine. Therefore, elucidation of the underlying etiology of hearing loss in newborns can have vast consequences and implications.

The first few years of life are critical for speech and language development. Before the implementation of newborn hearing screening, hearing loss in a large number of children remained un-

Table 1. Comparisons of traditional and next-generation newborn hearing screening

Hearing screening	Traditional	Next-generation
Method	OAE and ABR	OAE and ABR plus WGS
Type	phenotypic	phenotypic + genetic
Symptomatic	yes	not required
Prognostic	no	maybe
Accurate recurrence risk estimation	no	yes
Etiology	no	yes
Precision medicine	no	may inform
Cost	$10–50/baby, single purpose, stable	<$10,000/baby, life-time, decreasing
Turnaround time	immediately	days
Sensitivity	unable to detect later-onset cases	expected higher, validation ongoing
Specificity	transient loss as false positives	expected higher, validation ongoing

ABR = Auditory brainstem response test; OAE = otoacoustic emission test; WGS = whole-genome sequencing.

noticed until after they missed the critical period for language acquisition. Studies have shown that children with hearing loss who began receiving treatment at an early age demonstrated language skills that were comparable to their hearing peers, regardless of the degree of hearing loss. Children whose hearing loss was identified by 6 months of age and who received early intervention scored significantly higher in language skills and social emotional development than children whose hearing loss was identified after 6 months of age [38]. In addition, a 2006 study revealed that infants who begin remediation for their hearing loss before 6 months of age experience emotional and social development in parallel with their physical development. Researchers estimate that children who receive treatment early in life in the form of a cochlear implant can save $30,000–200,000 in special education costs by the time they graduate from high school because they are more likely to be placed into mainstream classrooms [39]. Since the adoption of universal newborn hearing screening in the United States and other parts of the world, many infants with congenital hearing loss have received diagnosis shortly after birth and benefited from early intervention programs by 6 months of age.

Traditional Newborn Hearing Screening

The History of Newborn Hearing Screening and Current Status

Newborn hearing screening has been universally adopted since the 1990s. Given its importance, the National Institutes of Health's Consensus Development Conference on Early Identification of Hearing Loss in 1993 concluded that all newborns should have hearing screening, preferably prior to hospital discharge. Technological advances made possible routine automated screening methods to test a baby's hearing. These tests include acoustical otoacoustic emission, which tests for an infant's cochlear function, and electrophysiological auditory brainstem response, which measures the electrical responses of the auditory system (table 1). Both methods are functional screening tests that directly assess a baby's auditory function at the moment of testing, but do not reveal the underlying etiology of a hearing disorder. At that time, only 11 hospitals screened more than 90% of babies born there. In 1997, an NIH-convened expert panel recommended standard screening methods for use in nationwide newborn hearing screening programs. The Congress passed the

Newborn and Infant Hearing Screening and Intervention Act of 1999, which was amended in 2010 to emphasize 'diagnosis' and to reauthorize through 2015. As of the date this article is written, the Act of 2015 to reauthorize the program has passed the House. With the Federal support, now every state and territory in the United States has established the Early Hearing Detection and Intervention program. Of these, 46 states plus the District of Columbia, Guam, and Puerto Rico have mandated newborn hearing screening programs and 38 offer early intervention [40].

Limitations of Current Functional Hearing Screening Methods

Conventional functional hearing screening tests have been widely used in current newborn hearing screening programs. However, there are some limitations (table 1). The screening results are not very accurate. These tests have a false positive rate over 75% in the initial hospital screening and require a follow-up confirmatory test [41], yet they only detect symptomatic hearing loss, thus missing up to 50% of educationally significant childhood hearing loss cases. The high false positive rate may be due to immaturity in preterm babies or temporary hearing impairment caused by fluid in the ear canals, which can resolve over time. Even with follow-up confirmatory tests and physical examination, clinical diagnosis often does not distinguish among different types of hearing loss. For those babies who have passed conventional newborn hearing screening but who may develop hearing loss later during early childhood, a false negative screening result may give the family a false sense of relief. Therefore, for babies with a family history of hearing loss, a follow-up auditory evaluation is recommended even if they pass the newborn hearing screening. This will entail significant medical cost that may be avoided if the genetic cause of hearing loss for the family is known and the newborn does not have it.

Current screening methods will not inform the family of the molecular etiology of hearing loss, which would be extremely useful for families. As mentioned earlier, an accurate genetic diagnosis for hereditary hearing loss will guide the choice of clinical management and assure timely intervention. Knowing a definitive diagnosis of hearing loss will also likely urge the family to be in compliance with the early intervention program. Furthermore, it will not only benefit the affected baby, but also the whole family. Genetic testing results can provide a prognosis of a baby's future development before the onset of the hearing loss. They can be used for families to estimate the risk of recurrence and to make informed reproductive planning.

Next-Generation Newborn Hearing Screening

Next-generation newborn hearing screening will incorporate genomic analysis in addition to the traditional phenotypic screening because genomic screening can overcome many of the limitations of current screening methods (table 1). It can elucidate the genetic etiology regardless of clinical manifestation, translating into opportunities for optimal management at the earliest possible time. At present, less than a handful of genetic variants are evaluated in newborns with abnormal functional hearing tests, far less than the growing number of genes known to be associated with hearing loss, many with largely different implications. Early detection and intervention of hearing loss before the critical period of speech and language acquisition translate into better intellect, social skills and quality of life. Thanks to high-throughput sequencing, 16% of currently known nonsyndromic hearing loss genes were discovered in the past 2 years, outpacing the development of gene-specific clinical diagnostic tests. These numbers strongly support a critical need for a clinical genomics application to identify the genetic and molecular etiology of hearing loss, which often presents in one general, and indistinguishable clinical diagnosis. A clinical genomic newborn hearing screen with greatly improved sensitivity, specificity, and clinical utility is urgently needed.

Genomic analyses will become routine to screen for all actionable genetic disorders including hereditary hearing loss in a newborn. Once genomic newborn screening is universally adopted, parental genomic information will be available for future generations. A newborn's genomic information will be compared to that of his/her parents. The genomic screening results will be used to identify genetic variants including small nucleotide variation, copy number variation, and structural variation in newborns. The data will be correlated with audiological screening to identify newborns with hearing loss and guide them for the most appropriate follow-up medical management plans.

In addition to genetic etiologies, hearing loss is recognized to arise from maternally acquired infections. By far the most common is congenital CMV infection. In one retrospective study of DNA extracted from newborn blood spots, 10% of infants with congenital hearing loss and 35% of those with moderate to severe late-onset loss had CMV infections at birth [1]. Though much less common, other prenatal infections such as rubella and toxoplasmosis can also result in hearing loss. By interrogating non-aligned sequences against the vast datasets of infectious genomes, genomic screening may gain new insights into unrecognized and potentially treatable or preventable causes of hearing loss.

Mature Next-Generation Technologies
Genomic analysis technologies such as whole-exome sequencing have been productively applied to the discovery of the etiology of rare single gene disorders and have provided clinical insight into the etiology of complex disorders [42–46]. Innovative genomic analysis approaches allow rapid screening for genetic causes of diseases. Exploiting the power of these approaches will bring

huge public health benefits as many genetic disorders may be prevented or treated before severe complications develop.

While the exome is enriched for clinically interpretable variants, coding variation accounts for only a subset of all pathogenic variants. Another major contributor is structural variants including copy number variants. New studies have shown that whole-genome sequencing (WGS) provides not only even coverage and better accuracy of variant calling in regions targeted by whole-exome sequencing [47], but can also identify genetic variants in noncoding regions, copy number variants, and structural variants [48, 49]. WGS can be completed within a couple of days [50].

Although next-generation sequencing has been offered as a clinical diagnostic test around the world [51–53], adoption of genomic newborn screening remains controversial due to cost, turnaround time and interpretation concerns as well as associated ethical, legal and social issues. Coupling genomic technologies with current newborn hearing screening and transforming it into a next-generation clinical newborn screening application is therefore a tremendous challenge, yet a worthy undertaking.

Affordable Next-Generation Genomic Newborn Hearing Screening
President Obama announced the Precision Medicine Initiative in his 2015 State of the Union Address and then proposed the cancer 'moonshot' in 2016. Accurate molecular diagnoses of diseases are the prerequisites of precision medicine, and baseline genetic makeups of the germline DNA of normal tissues in cancer patients are the 'launching pad' for the cancer 'moonshot'. Because germline genetic information does not change in each individual throughout the lifespan, one would only need to have a comprehensive genomic analysis once in his or her life. The best time for this 'once-in-a-life-time' test is undoubtedly during the newborn period.

The cost of next-generation newborn hearing screening is not as high as one may think. Newborn hearing screening has always been an integral part of newborn screening with other metabolic, genetic, and endocrine disorders. We envision that innovative genomic approaches will soon be translated into newborn molecular screening. Currently the test of a single pathogenic variant, for example the NM_004004:c.35delG pathogenic variant in *GJB2* for nonsyndromic hearing loss, costs several hundreds of dollars and a comprehensive panel of known hearing loss genes costs thousands of dollars. Because next-generation genomic screening can be applied to many different genetic disorders, the cost of the test can be shared by hearing loss and many other hereditary conditions. Clinical-grade WGS is currently available for less than $10,000 [54], a significant portion of which is for interpretation of the results. For a 'once-in-a-life-time' test, as hearing loss accounts for <1/100 of the conditions screened, the next-generation newborn hearing screening would cost less than 0.3 cents/day for an average lifespan of 70 years. With the continued decrease in the cost of sequencing and computing, and accumulation of knowledge that decreases the cost of variant interpretation, cost will no longer be a concern. Besides, the information generated from the screening program will bring invaluable knowledge. Therefore, next-generation genomic newborn hearing screening is predicted to become the routine of public health care in the future as the newborn screening program is today.

Socio-Economical and Public Health Impact
Next-generation genomic newborn hearing screening makes economical sense to society as a whole. Payers, mainly health insurance companies, have moved in the positive direction. In January 2016, Independence Blue Cross and NantHealth announced GPS Cancer, insurance coverage for a comprehensive whole genome and proteome molecular diagnostic platform, which was the first in the United States. As tumor-normal comparison is required, WGS test of normal tissue is also covered. According to the Centers for Disease Control and Prevention, about 4 million babies are born in the United States in a year, and the American Cancer Society estimates 1.7 million new cancer cases a year. Therefore, germline WGS analysis would have been covered in more than 40% of the US population for cancer diagnostic testing. Because somatic mutations occur throughout one's life, a sample from the newborn period would represent the best normal control. Furthermore, newborn genomic screening would leave the information in an individual's medical records available for other health care needs, such as blood group typing, pharmacogenetics risk assessment, carrier screening for reproductive planning, hence saving healthcare dollars in many ways.

New technologies have made gene therapy a promising new approach to the treatment of hearing loss. As of December 2015, at least 6 clinical trials have been underway on patients to test drug and gene therapies aimed at preventing or reversing hearing loss [55]. Because of the targeted nature of precision medicine, identification of targets is key to the success of these trials. Huge resources have been put into stratifying patients based on their genetic makeup. The results of next-generation genomic newborn hearing screening eliminate the need for these expensive and time-consuming patient screening tests, and will speed up the drug discovery and therapeutic validation processes.

Ethical Considerations of Next-Generation
Newborn Hearing Screening
Newborn screening is a mandatory public health service. Each state public health department decides the scope of the screening. A successful next-generation newborn hearing screening program must be built on the ground of the 4 principles of biomedical ethics: beneficence, non-maleficence, justice, and autonomy. We have discussed the benefits of next-generation genetic

screening to both individual families and to society as a whole, which has clearly demonstrated beneficence. However, genomic testing may also bring necessities of follow-up confirmatory tests, large amounts of indeterminate results, and possible psychosocial stress. Paradoxically, the knowledge distilled from big data through universal newborn screening will improve the accuracy and predictive values of genomic analysis results, which is the key to reduce these negative consequences. Therefore, non-maleficence lies in the ability of next-generation newborn screening to balance itself. As next-generation newborn hearing screening will be offered to each individual equally, it distributes health resources fairly to those who need treatment, thus satisfying the justice principle. Finally, to achieve autonomy, educational programs need to be in place to help the general public to understand the complexity of genomic analysis, and parents will be given the opportunity to make informed decisions regarding opting out of receiving certain results.

Conclusions

In summary, translating genomic analysis into the next-generation newborn hearing screening program will have significant public health impact. It is expected to elucidate the exact molecular etiology for hereditary hearing loss, which will enable more accurate diagnoses, better quality of care, more effective genetic counseling, as well as improved cost-effectiveness and reduced disparity in medical care. We anticipate clinical validity, clinical utility and acceptance of genomic screening to be established in clinical research studies soon, which will lead to solutions to overcome the cost and process barriers. In addition, we expect universal adoption of next-generation genomic newborn hearing screening will contribute significantly to genotype-phenotype studies, to establish a robust framework for assessing long-term clinical outcomes, and to provide empirical data for determining recurrence risks. Moreover, genomic screening in the population will contribute fundamental knowledge to our understanding of disease mechanisms and have profound public health implications. Insights from the big data accumulated from the next-generation genomic screening will broadly advance the use of genomics in clinical evaluations of other malformations, as many human syndromes including hearing loss as a clinical feature also affect another system. Genomic screening for genetic defects in hearing loss genes is but one application of the next-generation newborn health screening. In the new era of precision medicine, next-generation newborn screening results will inform physicians and family members about ameliorative strategies or ways to promote effective parental use of the information.

References

1 Barbi M, Binda S, Caroppo S, Ambrosetti U, Corbetta C, Sergi P: A wider role for congenital cytomegalovirus infection in sensorineural hearing loss. Pediatr Infect Dis J 2003;22:39–42.

2 Foulon I, Naessens A, Foulon W, Casteels A, Gordts F: A 10-year prospective study of sensorineural hearing loss in children with congenital cytomegalovirus infection. J Pediatr 2008;153:84–88.

3 Goderis J, De Leenheer E, Smets K, Van Hoecke H, Keymeulen A, Dhooge I: Hearing loss and congenital CMV infection: a systematic review. Pediatrics 2014;134:972–982.

4 Salviz M, Montoya JG, Nadol JB, Santos F: Otopathology in congenital toxoplasmosis. Otol Neurotol 2013;34:1165–1169.

5 Andrade GM, Resende LM, Goulart EM, Siqueira AL, Vitor RW, Januario JN: Hearing loss in congenital toxoplasmosis detected by newborn screening. Braz J Otorhinolaryngol 2008;74:21–28.

6 McLeod R, Boyer K, Karrison T, Kasza K, Swisher C, et al: Outcome of treatment for congenital toxoplasmosis, 1981–2004: The National Collaborative Chicago-Based, Congenital Toxoplasmosis Study. Clin Infect Dis 2006;42: 1383–1394.

7 Byl FM, Adour KK: Auditory symptoms associated with herpes zoster or idiopathic facial paralysis. Laryngoscope 1977;87:372–379.

8 Hopkins LA: Congenital deafness and other defects following German measles in the mother. Am J Dis Child 1946;72: 377–381.

9 Dobbin JM, Perkins JH: Otosyphilis and hearing loss: response to penicillin and steroid therapy. Laryngoscope 1983;93: 1540–1543.

10 Daneshi A, Ajalloueyan M, Ghasemi MM, Hashemi BS, Emamjome H, et al: Complications in a series of 4400 paediatric cochlear implantation. Int J Pediatr Otorhinolaryngol 2015;79:1401–1403.

11 Erenberg A, Lemons J, Sia C, Trunkel D, Ziring P: Newborn and infant hearing loss: detection and intervention. American Academy of Pediatrics. Task Force on Newborn and Infant Hearing, 1998–1999. Pediatrics 1999;103:527–530.

12 Hofkosh D, Thompson AE, Nozza RJ, Kemp SS, Bowen A, Feldman HM: Ten years of extracorporeal membrane oxygenation: neurodevelopmental outcome. Pediatrics 1991;87:549–555.

13 Mann T, Adams K: Sensorineural hearing loss in ECMO survivors. Extracorporeal membraneous oxygenation. J Am Acad Audiol 1998;9:367–370.

14 Prezant TR, Agapian JV, Bohlman MC, Bu X, Oztas S, et al: Mitochondrial ribosomal RNA mutation associated with both antibiotic-induced and non-syndromic deafness. Nat Genet 1993;4:289–294.

15 Xu H, Robinson GW, Huang J, Lim JY, Zhang H, et al: Common variants in *ACYP2* influence susceptibility to cisplatin-induced hearing loss. Nat Genet 2015;47:263–266.

16 Eppsteiner RW, Shearer AE, Hildebrand MS, Taylor KR, Deluca AP, et al: Using the phenome and genome to improve genetic diagnosis for deafness. Otolaryngol Head Neck Surg 2012;147:975–977.

17 Shearer AE, Smith RJ: Genetics: advances in genetic testing for deafness. Curr Opin Pediatr 2012;24:679–686.

18 Van Camp G, Smith RJ: Hereditary hearing loss homepage. Updated May 13, 2015. http://hereditaryhearingloss.org/.

19 HGNC: Hugo Gene Nomenclature Committee. http://www.genenames.org/.

20 McKusick VA: OMIM® – Online Mendelian inheritance in man. http://omim.org/.

21 Kelsell DP, Dunlop J, Stevens HP, Lench NJ, Liang JN, et al: Connexin 26 mutations in hereditary non-syndromic sensorineural deafness. Nature 1997;387: 80–83.

22 Morton CC, Nance WE: Newborn hearing screening – a silent revolution. N Engl J Med 2006;354:2151–2164.

23 Shargorodsky J, Curhan SG, Curhan GC, Eavey R: Change in prevalence of hearing loss in US adolescents. JAMA 2010; 304:772–778.

24 White KR, Forsman I, Eichwald J, Munoz K: The evolution of early hearing detection and intervention programs in the United States. Semin Perinatol 2010; 34:170–179.

25 Kenna MA: Medical management of childhood hearing loss. Pediatr Ann 2004;33:822–832.

26 Eppsteiner RW, Shearer AE, Hildebrand MS, Deluca AP, Ji H, et al: Prediction of cochlear implant performance by genetic mutation: the spiral ganglion hypothesis. Hear Res 2012;292:51–58.

27 Damen GW, van den Oever-Goltstein MH, Langereis MC, Chute PM, Mylanus EA: Classroom performance of children with cochlear implants in mainstream education. Ann Otol Rhinol Laryngol 2006;115:542–552.

28 Lalwani AK, Budenz CL, Weisstuch AS, Babb J, Roland JT Jr, Waltzman SB: Predictability of cochlear implant outcome in families. Laryngoscope 2009;119: 131–136.

29 Avraham KB: Rescue from hearing loss in Usher's syndrome. N Engl J Med 2013;369:1758–1760.

30 Lentz JJ, Jodelka FM, Hinrich AJ, McCaffrey KE, Farris HE, et al: Rescue of hearing and vestibular function by antisense oligonucleotides in a mouse model of human deafness. Nat Med 2013;19:345–350.

31 Maeda Y, Sheffield AM, Smith RJ: Therapeutic regulation of gene expression in the inner ear using RNA interference. Adv Otorhinolaryngol 2009;66:13–36.

32 Zuris JA, Thompson DB, Shu Y, Guilinger JP, Bessen JL, et al: Cationic lipid-mediated delivery of proteins enables efficient protein-based genome editing in vitro and in vivo. Nat Biotechnol 2015;33:73–80.

33 Stein EA, Dufour R, Gagne C, Gaudet D, East C, et al: Apolipoprotein B synthesis inhibition with mipomersen in heterozygous familial hypercholesterolemia: results of a randomized, double-blind, placebo-controlled trial to assess efficacy and safety as add-on therapy in patients with coronary artery disease. Circulation 2012;126:2283–2292.

34 Akil O, Seal RP, Burke K, Wang C, Alemi A, et al: Restoration of hearing in the VGLUT3 knockout mouse using virally mediated gene therapy. Neuron 2012;75: 283–293.

35 Chen W, Jongkamonwiwat N, Abbas L, Eshtan SJ, Johnson SL, et al: Restoration of auditory evoked responses by human ES-cell-derived otic progenitors. Nature 2012;490:278–282.

36 Golub JS, Tong L, Ngyuen TB, Hume CR, Palmiter RD, et al: Hair cell replacement in adult mouse utricles after targeted ablation of hair cells with diphtheria toxin. J Neurosci 2012;32:15093–15105.

37 Askew C, Rochat C, Pan B, Asai Y, Ahmed H, et al: *Tmc* gene therapy restores auditory function in deaf mice. Sci Transl Med 2015;7:295ra108.

38 Yoshinaga-Itano C: Early intervention after universal neonatal hearing screening: impact on outcomes. Ment Retard Dev Disabil Res Rev 2003;9:252–266.

39 Schnell-Inderst P, Kunze S, Hessel F, Grill E, Siebert U, et al: Screening of the hearing of newborns – update. GMS Health Technol Assess 2006;2:Doc20.

40 American Speech-Language Hearing Association: State overviews. http://www.asha.org/advocacy/state/info/.

41 Clemens CJ, Davis SA, Bailey AR: The false-positive in universal newborn hearing screening. Pediatrics 2000; 106:E7.

42 de Ligt J, Willemsen MH, van Bon BW, Kleefstra T, Yntema HG, et al: Diagnostic exome sequencing in persons with severe intellectual disability. N Engl J Med 2012;367:1921–1929.

43 Foo JN, Liu JJ, Tan EK: Whole-genome and whole-exome sequencing in neurological diseases. Nat Rev Neurol 2012;8: 508–517.

44 Hanchard NA, Murdock DR, Magoulas PL, Bainbridge M, Muzny D, et al: Exploring the utility of whole-exome sequencing as a diagnostic tool in a child with atypical episodic muscle weakness. Clin Genet 2013;83:457–461.

45 Rauch A, Wieczorek D, Graf E, Wieland T, Endele S, et al: Range of genetic mutations associated with severe non-syndromic sporadic intellectual disability: an exome sequencing study. Lancet 2012;380:1674–1682.

46 Yu Y, Wu BL, Wu J, Shen Y: Exome and whole-genome sequencing as clinical tests: a transformative practice in molecular diagnostics. Clin Chem 2012;58: 1507–1509.

47 Meienberg J, Bruggmann R, Oexle K, Matyas G: Clinical sequencing: is WGS the better WES? Hum Genet 2016;135: 359–362.

48 Dong Z, Zhang J, Hu P, Chen H, Xu J, et al: Low-pass whole-genome sequencing in clinical cytogenetics: a validated approach. Genet Med 2016, E-pub ahead of print.

49 Yuen RK, Thiruvahindrapuram B, Merico D, Walker S, Tammimies K, et al: Whole-genome sequencing of quartet families with autism spectrum disorder. Nat Med 2015;21:185–191.

50 Miller NA, Farrow EG, Gibson M, Willig LK, Twist G, et al: A 26-hour system of highly sensitive whole genome sequencing for emergency management of genetic diseases. Genome Med 2015;7:100.

51 Lee H, Deignan JL, Dorrani N, Strom SP, Kantarci S, et al: Clinical exome sequencing for genetic identification of rare Mendelian disorders. JAMA 2014; 312:1880–1887.

52 van Zelst-Stams WA, Scheffer H, Veltman JA: Clinical exome sequencing in daily practice: 1,000 patients and beyond. Genome Med 2014;6:2.

53 Yang Y, Muzny DM, Xia F, Niu Z, Person R, et al: Molecular findings among patients referred for clinical whole-exome sequencing. JAMA 2014;312: 1870–1879.

54 TruGenome Clinical Sequencing Services. www.illumina.com/clinical/illumina_clinical_laboratory/trugenome-clinical-sequencing-services.html.

55 ClinicalTrials.gov. A service of the U.S. National Institutes of Health. https://clinicaltrials.gov.

Cynthia C. Morton, PhD, FFACMG
Harvard Medical School Center for Hereditary Deafness
Brigham and Women's Hospital
Harvard Medical School
77 Avenue Louis Pasteur, NRB 160
Boston, MA 02115 (USA)
E-Mail cmorton@partners.org

Vona B, Haaf T (eds): Genetics of Deafness. Monogr Hum Genet. Basel, Karger, 2016, vol 20, pp 40–55
(DOI: 10.1159/000444564)

Clinical Challenges in Diagnosing the Genetic Etiology of Hearing Loss

Andrew C. Birkeland · Marci M. Lesperance

Division of Pediatric Otolaryngology, Department of Otolaryngology – Head and Neck Surgery, University of Michigan Health System, Ann Arbor, Mich., USA

Abstract

Tremendous progress has been made over the past 25 years in identifying genes responsible for nonsyndromic or syndromic deafness. However, clinical challenges remain that limit the number of patients for whom a genetic etiology can be determined. This chapter will address the diagnostic evaluation of patients with hearing loss, considering the audiological, radiological and clinical aspects.   © 2016 S. Karger AG, Basel

Background

Communicatively significant permanent hearing loss affects up to 1–3:1,000 newborns, with 50–60% of cases estimated to result from genetic etiologies [1]. Infectious diseases such as meningitis and congenital rubella have historically been a significant cause of childhood hearing loss, but these etiologies have declined in incidence due to successful immunization programs and other efforts at prevention. The risk of hearing loss due to ototoxicity may be moderated by substituting a safer alternative drug, careful monitoring of drug levels, or co-administration of other drugs [2].

Thus, the proportion of childhood hearing loss due to genetic causes is likely to increase, as medical advances reduce the incidence of hearing loss due to environmental causes.

It is helpful to categorize genetic hearing loss as syndromic (hearing loss accompanied by other clinical features) and nonsyndromic (isolated hearing loss). Overall, syndromic forms of hearing loss account for ~1/3 of genetic hearing loss, whereas nonsyndromic forms are responsible for 2/3 [3]. Inheritance patterns for nonsyndromic causes of hearing loss are autosomal dominant (20%), autosomal recessive (80%), or rarely X-linked (<1%) or mitochondrial (<1%) [1]. Mitochondrial and X-linked hearing loss may be more common than reported, as the hereditary nature of hearing loss might not be recognized in such families.

Since the identification of the first genes responsible for human deafness in the 1990s [4–6], there are now dozens of genes identified for nonsyndromic and syndromic deafness, and more yet to be discovered [7]. Indeed, deafness exemplifies genetic heterogeneity, and phenotypic characteristics are only somewhat helpful in identifying a genetic etiology. With the introduction and advancement of next-generation sequencing techniques, it is now possible to identify a genetic etiology in an increasing number of patients, and these technologies have facilitated the continued discovery of new genes [8].

The American College of Medical Genetics recommends evaluation by a geneticist for all children with permanent hearing loss [9]. Identifying the molecular genetic etiology of hearing loss is helpful to predict prognosis, guide treatment, identify potential comorbidities associated with a syndrome, and predict recurrence risk. However, the role of genetics consultation and genetic testing in the clinical evaluation for hearing loss continues to evolve. This chapter will focus on challenges to the current clinical evaluation and diagnosis of genetic hearing loss, as well as future directions in genetic testing for hearing loss. The otolaryngologist's expertise in the clinical evaluation of hearing loss may be very helpful to the clinician considering genetic testing of these patients.

Diagnostic Evaluation

Audiological Evaluation
In newborns, hearing is best evaluated by auditory brainstem response (ABR) during natural sleep. Behavioral audiometry can be used to evaluate hearing in infants who have reached a developmental age of ~6 months [10, 11]. Responses are elicited in the sound field, which reflect the better hearing ear, if a difference exists between ears. Thus, while localization ability can be assessed to some degree, a unilateral hearing loss cannot be ruled out by behavioral testing until the child is able to cooperate with ear-specific testing measures.

Pure tone audiometry with testing by air conduction and bone conduction is the gold standard to specify the degree of hearing loss, the frequencies affected, and the type of hearing loss (con-

ductive, sensorineural, or mixed). Confusion arises in the genetic literature when the type of hearing loss and frequencies affected are not described. Ideally, clinical reports would include the actual audiogram and document the manner of evaluation in order to allow the reader to interpret the results. In addition, the presence of any risk indicators for environmental or acquired hearing loss should be described.

It is difficult to specify the hearing loss phenotype with a particular gene given the variability that occurs even between individuals in the same family inheriting the same mutation (fig. 1). It is not uncommon for a large family to have at least 1 phenocopy, given the high incidence of hearing loss in the general population, but identifying the phenocopy among all the hearing impaired family members may be difficult. Adults may have an environmental component of hearing loss added on to the underlying genetic hearing loss, most commonly from noise exposure.

Types of Hearing Loss: Conductive and Sensorineural
Temporary or treatable causes of conductive hearing loss include Eustachian tube dysfunction, cerumen impaction, other disorders of the external auditory canal such as otitis externa, or disorders of the tympanic membrane such as perforation. Eustachian tube dysfunction inevitably accompanies cleft palate, which is itself a common feature of craniofacial syndromes. Prior otologic surgery or trauma should also be described. A minimal or mild low frequency conductive hearing loss is often seen after tympanostomy tube placement, and it may be difficult to detect a permanent source of conductive hearing loss until the patient's Eustachian tube dysfunction has resolved. A masking dilemma may make delineation of thresholds difficult in patients with bilateral mixed hearing loss.

Unlike temporary conductive hearing loss due to the causes discussed above, persistent conductive hearing loss should increase suspicion for a

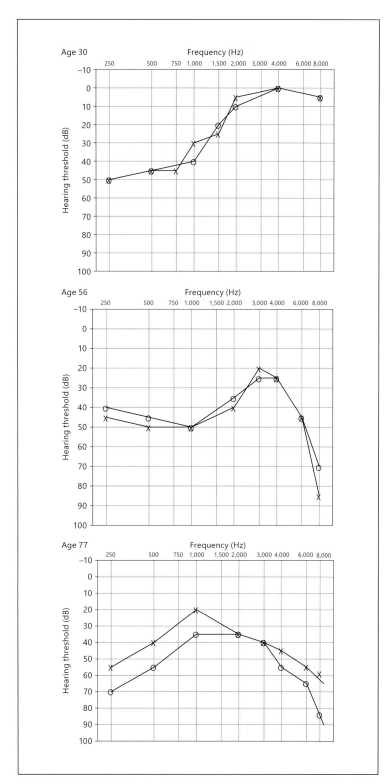

Fig. 1. Variability in hearing loss in 3 members of a family with the p.L829P mutation in *WFS1*. Note that low frequency SNHL is seen in all 3 individuals. However, with age, variability occurs in mid and high frequencies. Circles and X's indicate thresholds for right and left ears, respectively.

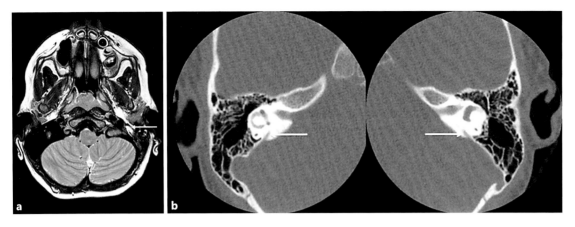

Fig. 2. Characteristic findings of enlarged vestibular aqueduct (arrows) on MRI (**a**) and CT (**b**).

genetic etiology. Otosclerosis is a form of progressive, delayed onset conductive hearing loss due to progressive fixation of the stapes. While otosclerosis is considered a genetic disease [12], no genes for otosclerosis have yet been identified. Congenital stapes ankylosis resulting in early onset maximum conductive hearing loss is a common feature of the *NOG* symphalangism syndromes [13]. Craniofacial syndromes are often associated with malformation or fixation of the ossicles, and/or external auditory canal atresia or stenosis. However, conductive hearing loss of genetic etiology is not necessarily permanent, as surgical procedures such as ossicular reconstruction or stapedotomy offer the possibility of improving or resolving conductive hearing loss.

Diagnostic challenges include 'inner ear conductive hearing loss,' manifested as conductive or mixed hearing loss despite an intact and mobile ossicular chain. Enlarged vestibular aqueduct syndrome (fig. 2) is the most common cause, typically manifesting as a low frequency conductive hearing loss and high frequency sensorineural hearing loss (SNHL) [14]. Superior semicircular canal dehiscence syndrome (fig. 3) may also present with a conductive component [15].

Finally, a wide spectrum of craniosynostosis syndromes are also associated with hearing loss, ranging from conductive hearing loss, which may be associated with cleft palate and/or ossicular malformations, to SNHL to mixed hearing loss. To add to the confusion, craniosynostosis with hearing loss such as Muenke syndrome is often referred to as 'nonsyndromic craniosynostosis.' Muenke syndrome results from a specific mutation in the *FGFR3* gene, p.P250R, and is characterized by low frequency SNHL and low penetrance craniosynostosis [16].

Auditory Neuropathy
Auditory neuropathy is defined as an absent or abnormal ABR with preserved outer hair cell function, as measured by otoacoustic emissions or by the cochlear microphonic response [17]. Auditory neuropathy is also referred to as auditory dys-synchrony, because the ABR measures the synchronous discharge of auditory nerve action potentials. More recently, the term 'auditory neuropathy spectrum disorder' has been used in an attempt to describe the heterogeneity of conditions which are associated with these audiological findings. These conditions include primary neuropathies of the auditory nerve (syndromic or nonsyndromic), cochlear nerve aplasia or hypoplasia, and synaptopathies of the inner hair cell, as is associated with *OTOF* mutations [18]. Neuro-

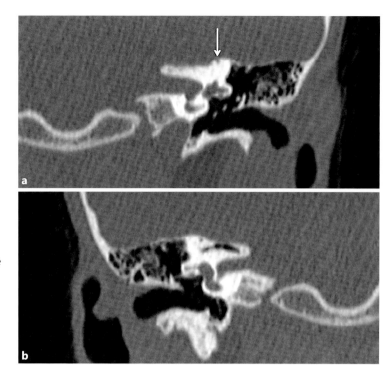

Fig. 3. Characteristic findings of superior semicircular canal dehiscence on CT of the temporal bone. **a** Left superior semicircular canal appears confluent with brain due to lack of bony covering (arrow). **b** Right superior semicircular canal with normal bony covering by way of comparison.

logical consultation should be considered in patients to rule out peripheral neuropathies, which may manifest years after onset of auditory symptoms.

To optimize detection of auditory neuropathy, patients with profound hearing loss should be evaluated with distortion product otoacoustic emissions (DPOAE) to assess for preservation of outer hair cell function. Middle ear dysfunction may cause a temporary loss of DPOAE responses, and thus it may be necessary to repeat DPOAE testing once middle ear pathology has resolved. ABR is the gold standard to diagnose auditory neuropathy, but it may require sedation or general anesthesia in children older than 3 months. Accurate diagnosis of auditory neuropathy is important, as it will prompt consideration of a different panel of genes than would be tested for SNHL. Likewise, the responsible genes for syndromic neuropathies are different from those that underlie nonsyndromic auditory neuropathy.

Onset of Hearing Loss
With the advent of ABR testing in the 1970s, newborn hearing screening began as high risk screening in infants with risk indicators for hearing loss. In the United States, universal newborn hearing screening was first implemented in Rhode Island in 1999, and became widespread following the 1999 Newborn and Infant Hearing Screening and Intervention Act. Currently, early hearing detection and intervention programs are in place across North America, Europe and Australia. In addition to newborn hearing screening, these programs include provisions for follow-up of children who are at risk for delayed onset or progressive hearing loss.

Identifying a hearing loss as congenital versus delayed onset is helpful to narrow the list of possible genes. However, challenges remain in identifying the specific age of onset of hearing loss. Firstly, newborn hearing screening is not completely 'universal,' as ~97% of newborns in the

United States receive hearing screenings [19]. Some states require only that a certain percentage of infants be screened, do not count parental refusals in the denominator, or require screening only by centers with a minimum number of births. In addition, babies born at home are less likely to have a newborn hearing screen. Secondly, screening methodologies and pass criteria vary widely, and thus a 'pass' on newborn hearing screening does not rule out hearing loss, particularly low frequency SNHL. Screening by DPOAE will miss children with auditory neuropathy or milder degrees of SNHL.

Close follow-up of children with a family history of hearing loss or risk indicators for delayed onset or progressive hearing loss is essential for early detection and intervention of hearing loss, regardless of newborn hearing screening results [20]. Many children with recessive nonsyndromic hearing loss will have a negative family history, and even some children with biallellic pathologic *GJB2* mutations may pass their newborn hearing screen [21, 22]. Expert panels continue to debate the value of adding genetic testing for common hearing loss genes such as *GJB2* to newborn screening panels [23].

School hearing screening programs vary across the United States, but hearing screenings are typically limited to the elementary school population (approximately age 12 years and under). Thus, it is difficult to determine the onset of hearing loss when it is first detected in adulthood. While it is likely that presbycusis has a genetic component, hearing loss in adults is more likely to have a monogenic etiology if it is early onset (prior to age 30 years).

History and Physical Exam
Identification of associated congenital abnormalities may indicate an underlying syndromic cause to hearing loss. The initial evaluation should include a robust family history to elicit inheritance patterns. Since the penetrance of hearing loss may be incomplete in some syndromes, it is helpful to inquire about specific syndromic features such as pigment alterations, kidney disease, or eye disease in other family members.

The history should also elicit any risk indicators for acquired hearing loss such as early prematurity, meningitis, birth trauma, neonatal jaundice, or prolonged neonatal intensive care unit stay [24]. However, these risk indicators may at times be 'red herrings', leading to false attribution of hearing loss to an acquired cause in patients ultimately discovered to have a genetic etiology. Perinatal exposure to ototoxic drugs or congenital infections should also be considered (see congenital human cytomegalovirus infection, below). In the absence of a definitive acquired cause, a genetic etiology of hearing loss should be considered, regardless of family history. In adults, environmental risk factors for hearing loss include occupational or recreational noise exposure, ototoxic drugs, and prescription drug abuse. The compounded effect of environmental hearing loss may cause difficulty in discerning any inheritance pattern in a family.

Otolaryngology evaluation includes performing a detailed otologic examination to identify auricular deformities such as microtia or preauricular pits, as well as external auditory canal atresia or stenosis. Assessment of the skull should include asymmetries that may suggest craniosynostosis, hemifacial microsomia, or macrocephaly. Specific syndromic features, such as those associated with Waardenburg syndrome (dystopia canthorum, white forelock), Pendred syndrome (euthyroid goiter), and branchio-oto-renal syndrome (preauricular or neck pits), among others, should be carefully noted.

Current guidelines recommend opthalmology examination, given the impact of vision loss on a patient with hearing loss [24]. Laboratory testing should be tailored to the individual patient, and there is no longer a role for 'shot-gun' laboratory testing to search for features of various syndromes.

Imaging

Imaging of the temporal bones is frequently obtained to assess inner and middle ear structures as well as the auditory nerve. The most commonly used modalities are computed tomography (CT) of the temporal bone and magnetic resonance imaging (MRI).

However, the majority of genetic causes are not associated with particular temporal bone anomalies, either because the defects are neuroepithelial and not morphogenetic, or because imaging has not been performed or reported for many rare types of genetic hearing loss.

CT will identify anatomic abnormalities in ~30% of cases of pediatric SNHL [25], including middle and inner ear dysplasias such as Mondini dysplasia. Intracranial calcifications suggest human cytomegalovirus (HCMV) or toxoplasmosis infections. An enlarged vestibular aqueduct will prompt genetic testing for *SLC26A4* mutations, which may segregate as nonsyndromic deafness [26] or as Pendred syndrome [27]. Mutations in *CHD7*, the gene that underlies CHARGE syndrome [28], are associated with dysplasias of the cochlea and semicircular canals, in particular the lateral (horizontal) semicircular canal [29].

The timing of imaging in relation to genetic testing continues to be debated, including the type of imaging. CT provides superior definition of the bony middle and inner ear structures, including the ossicles, cochlea and semicircular canals, but carries the risk of radiation to a young child [25]. In addition, a normal bony internal auditory canal on CT does not rule out an absent or small auditory nerve. MRI provides a higher diagnostic yield for unilateral or asymmetric hearing loss, but may also reveal incidental brain anomalies of uncertain significance that lead to parental distress without necessarily improving care [30]. MRI is superior at detection of aplasia and hypoplasia of the cochlear nerve, as well as tumors of the auditory nerve such as acoustic neuromas. MRI is also preferable to detect mild cochlear dysplasia and modiolar deficiencies.

Children may require sedation for imaging, adding the risk and expense of anesthesia. While an MRI avoids radiation, intravenous contrast is necessary, and the examination is typically longer, more expensive and more likely to require sedation. In summary, the cost-benefit ratio of imaging needs to be carefully weighed, particularly in comparison to genetic testing, as both investigations can be costly and inconclusive. Imaging is typically performed as part of the preoperative evaluation for cochlear implantation, but in milder cases of hearing loss may sometimes be deferred until children are old enough to cooperate without sedation. Progression of hearing loss will typically prompt imaging if it has not been previously performed.

Congenital Human Cytomegalovirus Infection

In developed countries, congenital HCMV infection is the most common nongenetic cause of early childhood hearing loss, occurring in up to 0.6% of births [31]. It is estimated to be responsible for up to 18% of early onset SNHL [32]. Up to 12% of infections are symptomatic, and carry up to a 40% risk for SNHL [32, 33]. However, SNHL is seen in up to 21% of otherwise asymptomatic congenital HCMV infections [34]. In order to differentiate congenital HCMV infection from postnatally acquired infection, diagnostic testing of blood, saliva or urine must be performed prior to age 3 weeks of life. However, a large proportion of cases have hearing loss that develops after the window of time to obtain HCMV testing [35]. There was some hope that newborn blood spots could be utilized for testing when hearing loss was diagnosed in older children, but unfortunately the sensitivity is inadequate [36].

Universal HCMV screening has been performed in some medical centers for years, and the value continues to be debated [33]. In 2013, the state of Utah passed a law requiring HCMV testing within 21 days of birth in all newborns who refer on 2 newborn hearing screenings. This law required a change in protocol to ensure that the hearing rescreen is done by age 14 days, instead of age 30 days as typically required. While there is evidence that antiviral therapy within the first 9 months of age has potential benefit [33], both oral valganciclovir and intravenous ganciclovir have side effects of bone marrow suppression. Thus, optimal management of asymptomatic HCMV infection remains to be determined, and the potential toxicities of antiviral treatment such as bone marrow suppression must be weighed against the potential for progressive hearing loss. The possibility of hearing loss due to congenital HCMV should be considered before embarking on more expensive genetic investigations such as whole-exome or whole-genome sequencing.

Diagnostic Challenges

Occult Features of Hearing Loss Syndromes
It is important to note that children and sometimes adults may present with hearing loss initially diagnosed as nonsyndromic, only to later develop features consistent with a syndrome. First of all, some features may not be present at birth or at the time that hearing loss is diagnosed. For example, the goiter in Pendred syndrome may not become apparent until adulthood [37]. Chromosomal deletions involving *STRC* and *CATSPER2* cause deafness and male infertility [38], another example of a comorbidity that may not be detected until adulthood. A syndrome may ultimately be diagnosed on a clinical basis when additional features become apparent, or through genetic testing that identifies a specific molecular etiology. Even if an initial genetics evaluation does not yield a unifying diagnosis, it is appropriate to refer back to the geneticist in a few years, as technology advances or if the patient develops new clinical problems.

Research participants may be ascertained in settings without prior examination by an expert clinician, or without available facilities to perform thorough clinical evaluation (such as pure tone audiometry or imaging). It may in fact be more cost-effective for research purposes to first perform linkage analysis rather than perform an exhaustive clinical examination [39]. For example, DFNB4 was initially classified as nonsyndromic deafness because the history of euthyroid goiter was not apparent [26]. The DFNB73 family members with apparent nonsyndromic deafness were found to have subclinical mild renal dysfunction detected after identifying mutations in a Bartter syndrome gene *(BSND)* [40].

Genetic testing is increasingly available and may be requested by an otolaryngologist, a primary care practitioner, or even by the patient himself. Thus, subtle features of syndromes may be missed in patients who have not been evaluated by an expert in dysmorphology. For example, CATSHL syndrome, which results from mutations in *FGFR3*, is characterized by hearing loss, tall stature and camptodactyly (fixed flexion deformity of the little finger) [41]. With the increasing use of multigene panels and whole-exome sequencing, patients may be more likely to have undergone a genetic test for a disorder such as Usher syndrome before (or in lieu of) a clinical evaluation for the syndrome. Thus, the thoroughness of the clinical evaluation and examination will determine the sensitivity for detection of syndromes.

'Missing' a syndrome has implications for genetic testing, since the responsible gene may not be included in the panel of genes tested. For example, at this time, the OtoSCOPE panel includes 109 genes for nonsyndromic deafness, as well as some genes responsible for syndromic deafness, including those underlying Usher and Pendred syndromes [42]. Given that there are over 400 hearing loss syndromes, it is not surprising that this panel does not include all genes responsible for syndromic hearing loss. Future re-

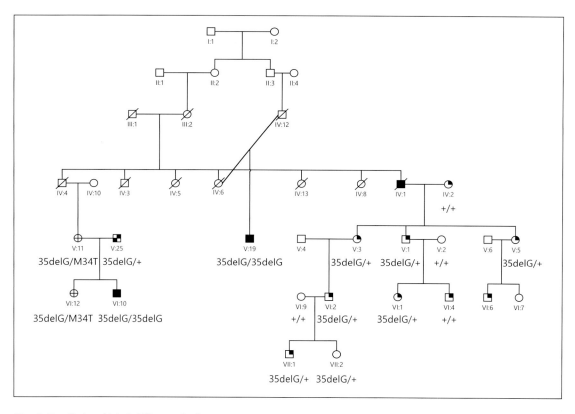

Fig. 4. Family in which 2 different deafness genes segregate. *GJB2* mutations cause recessive hearing loss in some individuals, but these mutations do not explain all cases of hearing loss. Note dominant hearing loss in the right-most branch originating from an individual who was initially presumed to have environmental hearing loss. Filled-in symbols = profound bilateral congenital SNHL; cross symbols = mild congenital SNHL; checkered symbols = phenocopy; black upper right quadrant = dominant progressive SNHL.

search should strive to identify syndromes that are both relatively common and more likely to be misdiagnosed as nonsyndromic hearing loss, such as the syndromes caused by *FGFR3* discussed above. Another gene worthy of consideration may be *CHD7*, as CHARGE syndrome is reported to have an incidence of 1 in 12,000 births [43], and some patients with CHARGE syndrome may appear to have isolated hearing loss. In particular, parent-to-child transmission of *CHD7* mutations has been reported, and the affected parent may manifest a mild form of CHARGE syndrome that is detected only after the child presents with classic features of the syndrome [44].

Bilineality and Pseudodominance

Bilineality refers to the presence of more than one gene for a condition segregating within a family. In some societies, assortative mating tends to occur among deaf individuals who meet at a school for the deaf, or due to linguistic homogamy, e.g. between a deaf person and a hearing individual who is fluent in sign language because of their deaf relatives [45]. Thus, it is not uncommon for more than one deafness gene to segregate within a family, particularly given the frequency of deafness due to *GJB2* mutations (fig. 4). In contrast, in other societies, marriages may be arranged based on ethnic or religious customs without regard to hearing loss. It is important to recognize the potential for

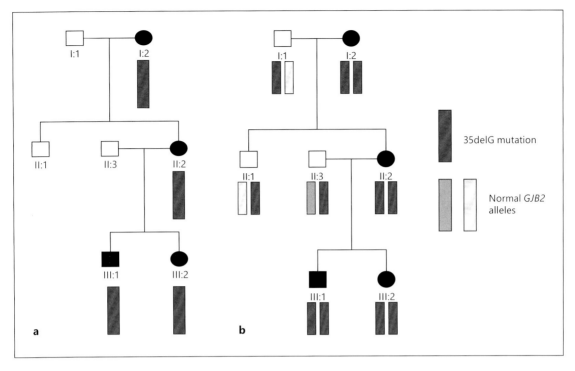

Fig. 5. Pseudodominance. **a** Hearing loss occurs in every generation, mimicking autosomal dominant inheritance, because the *GJB2* 35delG mutation is common in the general population. **b** Complete genotyping of all family members reveals recessive inheritance.

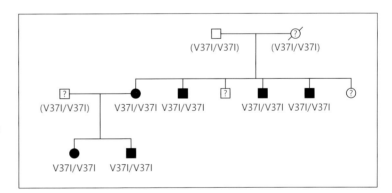

Fig. 6. Inheritance of hearing loss in a Thai-Laotian family mimics mitochondrial inheritance. Analysis of *GJB2* mutations reveals recessive inheritance.

multiple deafness genes within a kindred in order to properly determine the mode of inheritance.

Recessive hearing loss may be misdiagnosed as dominant (pseudodominance) (fig. 5) when a pathologic allele has a high frequency in the gen-eral population, such as 35delG in *GJB2* [46, 47]. Another example is the *GJB2* allele p.V37I, with an incidence of 8.5% in the Thai population [48], which may mimic pseudodominance or even ma-ternal inheritance (fig. 6).

Interpretation of Sequencing Results

In some instances, well-studied mutations are identified in a known deafness gene, allowing a definitive diagnosis of the genetic etiology of hearing loss. Novel mutations resulting in nonsense mutations such as stop codons or frameshifts may be reasonably predicted to be deleterious to gene function. A list of mutations and variants detected in patients with hearing loss is maintained in the Deafness Variation Database (http://deafnessvariationdatabase.org). However, many of these novel variants are designated at this time as variants of unknown significance. The significance of missense mutations and those occurring in splice sites, noncoding regions, or affecting post-transcriptional modification is particularly difficult to assess. While certain modeling programs (PolyPhen, SIFT) can provide clues as to the functional effects of specific mutations, they often disagree and are not fully predictive [49].

Given the large number of deafness genes, it is not infrequent that patients with recessive deafness are found to have a single pathologic mutation in a known deafness gene, or multiple deafness genes. Mutations in *SLC26A4* are the hallmark example. While Pendred syndrome is reliably associated with biallelic mutations [27], a significant proportion of patients with enlarged vestibular aqueduct syndrome have either 0 or 1 mutation in *SLC26A4*. It has been hypothesized that heterozygous mutations are sufficient to cause the phenotype, or that there are missing 'second alleles' that have not yet been discovered [50]. Digenic inheritance has also been proposed, but evidence is lacking to validate any of these hypotheses.

Another challenge is that databases of genetic variation are based on sequencing results from 'presumably' normal and healthy individuals without necessarily excluding individuals with hearing loss, or those who may develop hearing loss later in life. The significance of a very rare variant (0.1% or fewer of controls) is then difficult to interpret since the 'control' individual who contributed that DNA might actually have hearing loss. As more patients with hearing loss undergo genetic testing, the body of knowledge will increase and allow more accurate genotype-phenotype correlations, as has been elegantly performed for *GJB2* [51]. In addition, better assays of inner ear function are needed to provide a complementary approach to investigate the pathogenicity of novel variants.

Not surprisingly, there are currently over 100 genetic loci associated with nonsyndromic hearing loss, with no identified causative gene [52]. It is more difficult to identify the genetic etiology in dominant hearing loss, since all genes with a variation in a single copy must be considered; in recessive disorders, the pool of candidate genes may be restricted to those with mutations in both copies, a far smaller number. Identifying a second family of similar phenotype with a mutation in the same gene provides the strongest evidence [53], but family ascertainment remains the limiting factor. Modifier genes for deafness exist that can rescue the hearing loss phenotype, but these prove even more difficult to identify, likely again due to genetic heterogeneity [see chapter by Yousaf et al., this vol., pp. 73–83].

Ethical Considerations and Incidental Findings

Genetic testing for hearing loss carries the same potential for ethical issues common to all genetic testing, including paternity issues, incidental findings, balancing beneficence and autonomy, privacy, and providing 'clinically actionable' results [54]. Furthermore, ethical issues arise as to whether to extend such testing to fetuses [55, 56], and whether knowledge of hearing loss status can or should affect further care or considerations for future pregnancies. Consultation with geneticists and genetic counselors as well as ethicists and other experts will allow optimal counseling of the patient.

Genetic counseling based on haplotype-risk (linkage analysis) without identifying a gene mutation should be carried out with caution. The reliability of linkage analysis depends on the accuracy and availability of clinical information. Whereas a logarithm-of-odds (LOD) score >3.0 is typically the minimum threshold for linkage, a more conservative approach is to utilize a cut-off of 3.3 to correct for multiple comparisons. Indeed, analysis of some highly inbred families may yield more than one locus with a LOD score >3.0 [57]. The first locus for Usher syndrome type 1 was reported as mapping to chromosome 14, but the USH1A locus was later retracted when mutations in the USH1B gene, *MYO7A*, were identified in those families [58]. In another example, DFNA14 and DFNA6 were initially reported as 2 non-overlapping loci on chromosome 4p16 [59, 60]. Because of a phenocopy, the DFNA6 region was mis-specified, and it was later found that the DFNA6 and DFNA14 families had mutations in the same gene, *WFS1* [61].

Clinicians should weigh the risk of unintended or undesired discoveries versus the risk of not finding an answer. Although whole-exome/genome sequencing offers the potential for greater sensitivity, it adds the risk of incidental findings and the ethical issues inherent in whether to report such findings to patients. In patients who do undergo whole-exome/genome sequencing, the ramifications of identification and disclosure of incidental findings should be clearly discussed. The American College of Medical Genetics recommends evaluation of 57 'clinically-actionable' genes to be reported after exome/genome sequencing [62, 63].

Currently, there are no standard practices for disclosure of an incidental mutation in a hearing loss gene. If hearing loss is regarded in the same manner as a neurological condition for which there is no curative or preventative treatment, the conventional wisdom is against disclosure. However, in practice, a reasonable clinician may choose to disclose these findings, even if the onset of hearing loss is anticipated to occur in adulthood. Although hearing loss cannot be prevented or 'cured,' this knowledge may serve to prompt close monitoring of hearing so that intervention and rehabilitation may be offered as early as possible, and to help the individual make communication and vocational choices.

The Future of Genetic Testing for Hearing Loss

Expanding Genetic Causes of Hearing Loss
Screening panels will need to be continually updated to include newly discovered genes for nonsyndromic deafness, as well as the most common genes underlying syndromes that mimic nonsyndromic deafness. As more patients with hearing loss undergo genetic testing, and more genomes in the general population are sequenced, we will be able to better characterize rare variants as deafness-associated versus benign polymorphisms, with respect to various populations. Understanding how often a certain gene is mutated in various ethnic groups, as well as the frequency of specific mutations in each gene will be essential in order to tailor screening panels to specific populations [49, 64].

Viral gene therapy and antisense oligonucleotides have recently been demonstrated to restore hearing in mouse models [65, 66]. While such interventions are currently limited to animal models, it is anticipated that 'personalized medicine' for deafness will someday provide customized therapy according to the specific genetic etiology.

Mutations have been identified in noncoding regions of known deafness genes (such as *GJB2*), which result in loss of expression [67, 68], often occurring in compound heterozygosity with mutations in coding regions. The role of noncoding genetic regions in hereditary hearing loss is likely to grow in importance for the future. Noncoding regions include splice sites, promoters, enhancers, and other regulators of transcription. For example, a mutation in the 5′ untranslated region of *DIAPH3* leads to hearing loss through overexpression of the gene [69]. In addition, copy number variants (CNVs) have been demonstrated to be a cause of nonsyndromic hearing loss [70]. While some next-generation sequencing platforms can be specified to include detections of CNVs, CNVs may be missed by routine analysis.

Fidelity with large-scale sequencing can be an issue, with error rates across different platforms ranging from 0.1–15% [71]. Issues include difficulty with single base repeats, GC-rich motifs, and reads towards the $3'$ end of amplicons [72]. Additionally, the choice of an alignment and variant-calling program is important in order for sequenced genomes to be mapped correctly and to detect potential mutations versus benign polymorphisms. In unclear cases, traditional Sanger sequencing may be performed for verification. Next-generation sequencing platforms do allow for identification of DNA methylation, noncoding RNAs, and histone modifications [73]. However, the application of such technology is limited by our nascent understanding of the role of epigenetics in heritable hearing loss.

In order to go 'beyond the exomes,' methods other than traditional Sanger sequencing and whole-exome sequencing will be necessary to thoroughly evaluate intergenic and intragenic regions. However, it is more difficult to confirm the pathogenicity of such mutations in novel deafness genes, due to the inherent increased variation in these genomic regions. It is likely that whole-genome sequencing will be increasingly applied for cases of hearing loss in which whole-exome sequencing does not reveal an etiology. As noted above, it will be essential to exclude congenital HCMV infection and other environmental etiologies before widespread implementation of whole-genome sequencing.

Gene Expression

The inner ear represents the last frontier of gene expression. The proteins comprising the inner ear are present in minute quantities, and it is difficult to obtain human inner ear tissue in an ethical manner. Major gene expression databases such as BioGPS include a wide variety of human tissue types, including retina and several different brain regions, but do not include the cochlea or vestibular system [74]. Animal models have been very useful to help catalog the genes expressed in the inner ear, but typically reflect only one time point, such as P0, or one portion of the cochlea, such as the stereociliary bundle. The future will no doubt reveal many novel transcripts that are specific to the inner ear in general, or to the human inner ear in particular, either due to alternative splicing or to unique exons that are yet undiscovered within large introns. Likewise, better assays to characterize the functional effect of potentially disease-causing mutations in the cochlea must be developed in order to verify newly discovered genes.

Conclusion

Genetic testing for hearing loss has advanced greatly over the past 2 decades. Currently, over 100 genes have been identified for nonsyndromic hearing loss, and this list continues to expand. However, significant challenges remain in regards to clinical diagnosis as well as interpretation and identification of causative mutations. The importance of early intervention and the contributions of new technologies such as digital hearing aids and cochlear implants are universally recognized. However, we must acknowledge that our therapeutic options today involve rehabilitation and not prevention or cure of hearing loss. Ultimately, as our precision with identifying causative mutations improves, and as costs for genetic panels and genome sequencing decrease, genetic testing will undoubtedly be incorporated earlier and more frequently in the evaluation of hearing loss. Improving the ability to diagnose a molecular etiology of hearing loss will be a necessary step toward personalized medicine with therapies tailored to the genetic etiology.

References

1 Marazita ML, Ploughman LM, Rawlings B, Remington E, Arnos KS, Nance WE: Genetic epidemiological studies of early-onset deafness in the U.S. school-age population. Am J Med Genet 1993;46: 486–491.

2 Sha SH, Qiu JH, Schacht J: Aspirin to prevent gentamicin-induced hearing loss. N Engl J Med 2006;354:1856–1857.

3 Morton NE: Genetic epidemiology of hearing impairment. Ann N Y Acad Sci 1991;630:16–31.

4 de Kok YJ, van der Maarel SM, Bitner-Glindzicz M, Huber I, Monaco AP, et al: Association between X-linked mixed deafness and mutations in the POU domain gene POU3F4. Science 1995;267: 685–688.

5 Kelsell DP, Dunlop J, Stevens HP, Lench NJ, Liang JN, et al: Connexin 26 mutations in hereditary non-syndromic sensorineural deafness. Nature 1997;387: 80–83.

6 Lynch ED, Lee MK, Morrow JE, Welcsh PL, Leon PE, King MC: Nonsyndromic deafness DFNA1 associated with mutation of a human homolog of the Drosophila gene diaphanous. Science 1997; 278:1315–1318.

7 Smith RJH, Shearer AE, Hildebrand MS, Van Camp G: Deafness and hereditary hearing loss overview; in Pagon RA, Adam MP, Ardinger HH, Wallace SE, Amemiya A, et al (eds): GeneReviews® [Internet]. Seattle, University of Washington, 1993–2015 (February 14, 1999; updated January 9, 2014).

8 Vona B, Nanda I, Hofrichter MA, Shehata-Dieler W, Haaf T: Non-syndromic hearing loss gene identification: a brief history and glimpse into the future. Mol Cell Probes 2015;29:260–270.

9 Alford RL, Arnos KS, Fox M, Lin JW, Palmer CG, et al: American College of Medical Genetics and Genomics guideline for the clinical evaluation and etiologic diagnosis of hearing loss. Genet Med 2014;16:347–355.

10 Gravel JS, Wallace IF: Effects of otitis media with effusion on hearing in the first 3 years of life. J Speech Lang Hear Res 2000;43:631–644.

11 Sabo DL, Paradise JL, Kurs-Lasky M, Smith CG: Hearing levels in infants and young children in relation to testing technique, age group, and the presence or absence of middle-ear effusion. Ear Hear 2003;24:38–47.

12 Morrison AW: Genetic factors in otosclerosis. Ann R Coll Surg Engl 1967;41: 202–237.

13 Potti TA, Petty EM, Lesperance MM: A comprehensive review of reported heritable noggin-associated syndromes and proposed clinical utility of one broadly inclusive diagnostic term: NOG-related-symphalangism spectrum disorder (NOG-SSD). Hum Mutat 2011;32:877–886.

14 Valvassori GE: The large vestibular aqueduct and associated anomalies of the inner ear. Otolaryngol Clin North Am 1983;16:95–101.

15 Minor LB, Solomon D, Zinreich JS, Zee DS: Sound- and/or pressure-induced vertigo due to bone dehiscence of the superior semicircular canal. Arch Otolaryngol Head Neck Surg 1998;124:249–258.

16 Muenke M, Gripp KW, McDonald-McGinn DM, Gaudenz K, Whitaker LA, et al: A unique point mutation in the fibroblast growth factor receptor 3 gene (FGFR3) defines a new craniosynostosis syndrome. Am J Hum Genet 1997;60: 555–564.

17 Starr A, Picton TW, Sininger Y, Hood LJ, Berlin CI: Auditory neuropathy. Brain 1996;119:741–753.

18 Varga R, Kelley PM, Keats BJ, Starr A, Leal SM, et al: Non-syndromic recessive auditory neuropathy is the result of mutations in the otoferlin (OTOF) gene. J Med Genet 2003;40:45–50.

19 Gaffney M, Eichwald J, Gaffney C, Alam S; Centers for Disease Control and Prevention (CDC): Early hearing detection and intervention among infants – hearing screening and follow-up survey, United States, 2005–2006 and 2009–2010. MMWR Surveill Summ 2014; 63(suppl 2):20–26.

20 Young NM, Reilly BK, Burke L: Limitations of universal newborn hearing screening in early identification of pediatric cochlear implant candidates. Arch Otolaryngol Head Neck Surg 2011;137: 230–234.

21 Bitner-Glindzicz M: Hereditary deafness and phenotyping in humans. Br Med Bull 2002;63:73–94.

22 Green GE, Smith RJ, Bent JP, Cohn ES: Genetic testing to identify deaf newborns. JAMA 2000;284:1245.

23 Linden Phillips L, Bitner-Glindzicz M, Lench N, Steel KP, Langford C, et al: The future role of genetic screening to detect newborns at risk of childhood-onset hearing loss. Int J Audiol 2013;52:124–133.

24 American Academy of Pediatrics, Joint Committee on Infant Hearing: Year 2007 position statement: principles and guidelines for early hearing detection and intervention programs. Pediatrics 2007;120:898–921.

25 Chen JX, Kachniarz B, Shin JJ: Diagnostic yield of computed tomography scan for pediatric hearing loss: a systematic review. Otolaryngol Head Neck Surg 2014;151:718–739.

26 Li XC, Everett LA, Lalwani AK, Desmukh D, Friedman TB, et al: A mutation in PDS causes non-syndromic recessive deafness. Nat Genet 1998;18:215–217.

27 Everett LA, Glaser B, Beck JC, Idol JR, Buchs A, et al: Pendred syndrome is caused by mutations in a putative sulphate transporter gene (PDS). Nat Genet 1997;17:411–422.

28 Vissers LE, van Ravenswaaij CM, Admiraal R, Hurst JA, de Vries BB, et al: Mutations in a new member of the chromodomain gene family cause CHARGE syndrome. Nat Genet 2004;36:955–957.

29 Tellier AL, Cormier-Daire V, Abadie V, Amiel J, Sigaudy S, et al: CHARGE syndrome: report of 47 cases and review. Am J Med Genet 1998;76:402–409.

30 McClay JE, Booth TN, Parry DA, Johnson R, Roland P: Evaluation of pediatric sensorineural hearing loss with magnetic resonance imaging. Arch Otolaryngol Head Neck Surg 2008;134:945–952.

31 Kenneson A, Cannon MJ: Review and meta-analysis of the epidemiology of congenital cytomegalovirus (CMV) infection. Rev Med Virol 2007;17:253–276.

32 Goderis J, De Leenheer E, Smets K, Van Hoecke H, Keymeulen A, Dhooge I: Hearing loss and congenital CMV infection: a systematic review. Pediatrics 2014;134:972–982.

33 Cannon MJ, Griffiths PD, Aston V, Rawlinson WD: Universal newborn screening for congenital CMV infection: what is the evidence of potential benefit? Rev Med Virol 2014;24:291–307.

34 Foulon I, Naessens A, Foulon W, Casteels A, Gordts F: A 10-year prospective study of sensorineural hearing loss in children with congenital cytomegalovirus infection. J Pediatr 2008;153:84–88.

35 Dahle AJ, Fowler KB, Wright JD, Boppana SB, Britt WJ, Pass RF: Longitudinal investigation of hearing disorders in children with congenital cytomegalovirus. J Am Acad Audiol 2000;11:283–290.

36 Boppana SB, Ross SA, Novak Z, Shimamura M, Tolan RW Jr, et al: Dried blood spot real-time polymerase chain reaction assays to screen newborns for congenital cytomegalovirus infection. JAMA 2010;303:1375–1382.

37 Reardon W, Coffey R, Chowdhury T, Grossman A, Jan H, et al: Prevalence, age of onset, and natural history of thyroid disease in Pendred syndrome. J Med Genet 1999;36:595–598.

38 Vona B, Hofrichter MA, Neuner C, Schröder J, Gehrig A, et al: DFNB16 is a frequent cause of congenital hearing impairment: implementation of STRC mutation analysis in routine diagnostics. Clin Genet 2015;87:49–55.

39 Friedman TB, Rehman AU, Jenkinson E, Rehman AU, Morell RJ, et al: How much of nonsyndromic deafness is actually syndromic? Abstract presented at the 9th Molecular Biology of Hearing and Deafness Conference Stanford, CA, June 23, 2013. https://mbhd2013.stanford.edu/wp-content/uploads/2013/02/Program-MBHD_FINAL.pdf.

40 Riazuddin S, Anwar S, Fischer M, Ahmed ZM, Khan SY, et al: Molecular basis of DFNB73: mutations of BSND can cause nonsyndromic deafness or Bartter syndrome. Am J Hum Genet 2009;85:273–280.

41 Toydemir RM, Brassington AE, Bayrak-Toydemir P, Krakowiak PA, Jorde LB, et al: A novel mutation in FGFR3 causes camptodactyly, tall stature, and hearing loss (CATSHL) syndrome. Am J Hum Genet 2006;79:935–941.

42 Shearer AE, DeLuca AP, Hildebrand MS, Taylor KR, Gurrola J 2nd, et al: Comprehensive genetic testing for hereditary hearing loss using massively parallel sequencing. Proc Natl Acad Sci U S A 2010;107:21104–21109.

43 Källén K, Robert E, Mastroiacovo P, Castilla EE, Källén B: CHARGE association in newborns: a registry-based study. Teratology 1999;60:334–343.

44 Jongmans MC, Hoefsloot LH, van der Donk KP, Admiraal RJ, Magee A, et al: Familial CHARGE syndrome and the CHD7 gene: a recurrent missense mutation, intrafamilial recurrence and variability. Am J Med Genet A 2008; 146A:43–50.

45 Nance WE, Kearsey MJ: Relevance of connexin deafness (DFNB1) to human evolution. Am J Hum Genet 2004;74: 1081–1087.

46 Green GE, Scott DA, McDonald JM, Woodworth GG, Sheffield VC, Smith RJ: Carrier rates in the midwestern United States for GJB2 mutations causing inherited deafness. JAMA 1999;281:2211–2216.

47 Zelante L, Gasparini P, Estivill X, Melchionda S, D'Agruma L, et al: Connexin26 mutations associated with the most common form of non-syndromic neurosensory autosomal recessive deafness (DFNB1) in Mediterraneans. Hum Mol Genet 1997;6:1605–1609.

48 Wattanasirichaigoon D, Limwongse C, Jariengprasert C, Yenchitsomanus PT, Tocharoenthanaphol C, et al: High prevalence of V37I genetic variant in the connexin-26 (GJB2) gene among non-syndromic hearing-impaired and control Thai individuals. Clin Genet 2004; 66:452–460.

49 Shearer AE, Eppsteiner RW, Booth KT, Ephraim SS, Gurrola J 2nd, et al: Utilizing ethnic-specific differences in minor allele frequency to recategorize reported pathogenic deafness variants. Am J Hum Genet 2014;95:445–453.

50 Choi BY, Madeo AC, King KA, Zalewski CK, Pryor SP, et al: Segregation of enlarged vestibular aqueducts in families with non-diagnostic SLC26A4 genotypes. J Med Genet 2009;46:856–861.

51 Snoeckx RL, Huygen PL, Feldmann D, Marlin S, Denoyelle F, et al: GJB2 mutations and degree of hearing loss: a multicenter study. Am J Hum Genet 2005; 77:945–957.

52 Shearer AE, Smith RJ: Genetics: advances in genetic testing for deafness. Curr Opin Pediatr 2012;24:679–686.

53 Botstein D, Risch N: Discovering genotypes underlying human phenotypes: past successes for Mendelian disease, future approaches for complex disease. Nat Genet 2003;33(suppl):228–237.

54 Ross LF, Saal HM, David KL, Anderson RR: Technical report: ethical and policy issues in genetic testing and screening of children. Genet Med 2013;15:234–245.

55 Arnos KS: The implications of genetic testing for deafness. Ear Hear 2003;24: 324–331.

56 Ryan M, Miedzybrodzka Z, Fraser L, Hall M: Genetic information but not termination: pregnant women's attitudes and willingness to pay for carrier screening for deafness genes. J Med Genet 2003;40:e80.

57 Chen A, Wayne S, Bell A, Ramesh A, Srisailapathy CR, et al: New gene for autosomal recessive non-syndromic hearing loss maps to either chromosome 3q or 19p. Am J Med Genet 1997;71:467–471.

58 Gerber S, Bonneau D, Gilbert B, Munnich A, Dufier JL, et al: USH1A: chronicle of a slow death. Am J Hum Genet 2006;78:357–359.

59 Lesperance MM, Hall JW 3rd, Bess FH, Fukushima K, Jain PK, et al: A gene for autosomal dominant nonsyndromic hereditary hearing impairment maps to 4p16.3. Hum Mol Genet 1995;4:1967–1972.

60 Van Camp G, Kunst H, Flothmann K, McGuirt W, Wauters J, et al: A gene for autosomal dominant hearing impairment (DFNA14) maps to a region on chromosome 4p16.3 that does not overlap the DFNA6 locus. J Med Genet 1999; 36:532–536.

61 Bespalova IN, Van Camp G, Bom SJ, Brown DJ, Cryns K, et al: Mutations in the Wolfram syndrome 1 gene (WFS1) are a common cause of low frequency sensorineural hearing loss. Hum Mol Genet 2001;10:2501–2508.

62 ACMG Board of Directors: ACMG policy statement: updated recommendations regarding analysis and reporting of secondary findings in clinical genome-scale sequencing. Genet Med 2015;17:68–69.

63 Green RC, Berg JS, Grody WW, Kalia SS, Korf BR, et al: ACMG recommendations for reporting of incidental findings in clinical exome and genome sequencing. Genet Med 2013;15:565–574.

64 Chang MY, Choi BY: Strategy for the customized mass screening of genetic sensorineural hearing loss in Koreans. Korean J Audiol 2014;18:45–49.

65 Akil O, Seal RP, Burke K, Wang C, Alemi A, et al: Restoration of hearing in the VGLUT3 knockout mouse using virally mediated gene therapy. Neuron 2012;75: 283–293.

66 Lentz JJ, Jodelka FM, Hinrich AJ, McCaffrey KE, Farris HE, et al: Rescue of hearing and vestibular function by antisense oligonucleotides in a mouse model of human deafness. Nat Med 2013;19:345–350.

67 Rodriguez-Paris J, Tamayo ML, Gelvez N, Schrijver I: Allele-specific impairment of *GJB2* expression by *GJB6* deletion del(*GJB6*-D13S1854). PLoS One 2011;6:e21665.

68 Wilch E, Azaiez H, Fisher RA, Elfenbein J, Murgia A, et al: A novel DFNB1 deletion allele supports the existence of a distant *cis*-regulatory region that controls *GJB2* and *GJB6* expression. Clin Genet 2010;78:267–274.

69 Schoen CJ, Emery SB, Thorne MC, Ammana HR, Sliwerska E, et al: Increased activity of *Diaphanous homolog 3 (DIAPH3)/diaphanous* causes hearing defects in humans with auditory neuropathy and in *Drosophila*. Proc Natl Acad Sci U S A 2010;107:13396–13401.

70 Shearer AE, Kolbe DL, Azaiez H, Sloan CM, Frees KL, et al: Copy number variants are a common cause of non-syndromic hearing loss. Genome Med 2014; 6:37.

71 Xuan J, Yu Y, Qing T, Guo L, Shi L: Next-generation sequencing in the clinic: promises and challenges. Cancer Lett 2013;340:284–295.

72 Ulahannan D, Kovac MB, Mulholland PJ, Cazier JB, Tomlinson I: Technical and implementation issues in using next-generation sequencing of cancers in clinical practice. Br J Cancer 2013; 109:827–835.

73 Mensaert K, Denil S, Trooskens G, Van Criekinge W, Thas O, De Meyer T: Next-generation technologies and data analytical approaches for epigenomics. Environ Mol Mutagen 2014;55:155–170.

74 Wu C, Orozco C, Boyer J, Leglise M, Goodale J, et al: BioGPS: an extensible and customizable portal for querying and organizing gene annotation resources. Genome Biol 2009;10:R130.

Marci M. Lesperance, MD, FACS
Division of Pediatric Otolaryngology
Department of Otolaryngology – Head and Neck Surgery
University of Michigan Health System
CW-5-702, SPC 4241, 1540 East Hospital Drive
Ann Arbor, MI 48109-4241 (USA)
E-Mail lesperan@umich.edu

Vona B, Haaf T (eds): Genetics of Deafness. Monogr Hum Genet. Basel, Karger, 2016, vol 20, pp 56–72
(DOI: 10.1159/000444599)

Genetic Elucidation of Nonsyndromic Hearing Loss in the High-Throughput Sequencing Era

Barbara Vona[a] · Michaela A.H. Hofrichter[a] · Barry A. Chioza[b] · Andrew H. Crosby[b] · Indrajit Nanda[a] · Thomas Haaf[a]

[a]Institute of Human Genetics, Biocentre, Julius-Maximilians-University, Würzburg, Germany; [b]Molecular Genetics, RILD Institute, University of Exeter, Royal Devon and Exeter NHS Hospital, Wonford, Exeter, United Kingdom

Abstract

Hereditary hearing loss is a classic genetically heterogeneous condition with nearly 100 nonsyndromic hearing loss genes currently described and many more awaiting discovery. Priorities in the field with potentially rapid clinical application are the identification of all genes involved in the biological mechanisms of hearing and understanding their coordinated molecular interplay for normal auditory and nervous system functioning. Much of this momentum has been hindered by the inherent complexities of the genetics underlying deafness, as well as constraints such as requirements of large families for successful positional cloning. Major technological advancements in the past decade have empowered high-throughput next-generation sequencing approaches that have already facilitated the recognition of over 30 genes since 2010 and shifted hurdles away from achieving economical and time-efficient data toward accurate variant prioritization. Progress in the field of molecular genetics has never occurred at such a remarkable pace or been at such an exciting crossroad for expedited identification of the genes involved in hearing loss.   © 2016 S. Karger AG, Basel

One of the first notions in the literature referring to a hereditary background for hearing loss surfaced in the 16th century when the physician Johannes Schenck described a family in which several children presented profound congenital hearing loss despite having normal hearing parents. This observation was extended by Sir William Wilde in the mid-1800s to include the description of different inheritance patterns of deafness and a male-biased sex ratio among the congenitally deaf [1]. Unlike the times in which these 2 physicians lived, it is now understood that hearing loss is a heritable Mendelian trait. In fact, it is estimated that at least 50–60% of childhood hearing loss is due to a genetic aetiology [2]. Furthermore, it is clear that the pedigree described by Johannes Schenck was autosomal recessive, an inherited form of deafness comprising the largest fraction of genetic hearing loss (75–80% of cases), with autosomal dominant (20%), X-linked (2–5%), and mitochondrial (1%) forms recognized [3].

Table 1. Classifications of hearing loss

Classification	Description of hearing loss
Etiology	environmental/acquired (40–50%) or genetic (at least 50–60%)
Symmetry/laterality	bilateral (60–70%) or unilateral (30–40%)
Additional abnormalities	syndromic (30%) or nonsyndromic (70%)
Inheritance	recessive (75–80%), dominant (20%), X-linked (2–5%) or mitochondrial (1%)
Age of onset	congenital (present at birth), prelingual (0–5 years of age), postlingual (>5 years of age)
Type	sensorineural, conductive, mixed, central auditory dysfunction
Severity	mild (20–40 dB), moderate (41–55 dB), moderately severe (56–70 dB), severe (71–90 dB), profound (>90 dB)
Tone frequency affected	low (<1 kHz), middle (1–2 kHz), high (>2 kHz)
Progression	progressive or stable
Vestibular disorder	hearing loss associated with or without vestibular dysfunction

Characteristics for describing hearing loss [2, 3, 59].

Hearing loss is the most common sensory disorder in humans that affects 1.33 per 1,000 newborns with bilateral sensorineural hearing loss ≥40 decibels (dB) and increases throughout childhood to a rate of approximately 3.5 per 1,000 during adolescence [2]. Hearing loss can be described by virtue of symmetry, age of onset, anatomical site damaged, severity, and frequencies that are affected, as well as presence or absence of progression and vestibular disorder (table 1). Roughly 40–50% of hearing loss is nongenetic congenital or acquired with many affected neonates positive for risk factors and birth complications such as low birth weight, low APGAR (appearance, pulse, grimace response, activity, respiration) scores, hyperbilirubinemia or hypothyroidism [4]. Although this chapter will focus exclusively on the genetics of nonsyndromic hearing loss (NSHL), the nongenetic contributions to deafness are still far too great to neglect, despite the effectiveness of public health measures such as global immunization programs and improved pre- and neonatal care. Acquired forms of hearing loss occurring at any age arise from acoustic trauma, chronic otitis media, ototoxic medication exposure, wax or foreign body blockage of the ear canal, and head trauma. TORCH (toxoplasmosis, others, rubella, cytomegalovirus, and herpes simplex viruses) and other infectious diseases remain important nongenetic causes of hearing loss in neonates (table 2) [3].

Inherited forms of deafness can be further categorized into syndromic and nonsyndromic subgroups accounting for approximately 30 and 70% of all genetic forms, respectively. Nonsyndromic deafness is defined by isolated hearing loss, whereas syndromic deafness occurs in conjunction with other organ system abnormalities. One potential complexity with hearing-associated syndromes is the delayed presentation of additional clinical features that complicate successful differential diagnosis [5]. Paying careful attention to family history, audiological assessment, advanced diagnostic imaging, and comprehensive health workup are important for monitoring and surveillance of possible syndromes for the initiation of the appropriate therapy [5]. Early diagnosis of syndromic hearing loss is especially important to guide family and healthcare team decisions to reduce possible complications and support accurate preconception genetic counselling for parents wanting additional children [5], reiterating the predictive

Table 2. Common causes of hearing loss due to infectious disease

Pathogen	Vaccine	Treatment	Estimated prevalence at birth	Incidence of HL	Reference
Congenital					
CMV	no	intravenous ganciclovir or oral valganciclovir	up to 2%	21–24%	[2, 60]
LCMV	no	ribavirin, favipiravir	ND	7.4%	[61]
Rubella	yes	none	0% with vaccination series but still endemic in parts of the world	58%	[61]
Toxoplasma gondii	no	pyrimethamine/sulfadiazine, but generally not needed unless infection persists	1–10/10,000	as high as 28% in seropositive children	[62, 63]
Treponema pallidum	no	antibiotics	0.005–0.4%	3%	[4]
Congenital and acquired					
HIV	no	HAART	prevalence highly variable	22.5–33.5%	[61]
HSV types 1 and 2	no	acyclovir and prednisone	type 1: 1/2,000 to 1/8,000 type 2: 5.9/100,000	type 1: 4% among IgM-positive infants and children; type 2: 0.1% among IgM-positive infants and children	[61, 64]
Acquired					
Borrelia burgdorferi	no	antibiotics	NA	12%	[65]
Haemophilus influenzae type b	yes	antibiotics	NA	~6%	[66]
Measles	yes	supportive care	transmission occurs in childhood; infects susceptible children in epidemics; eliminated in many parts of the world due to immunization but still endemic in parts of the world	prior to widespread vaccination, measles accounted for 5–10% of profound HL; current estimates are 0.1–3.4%	[61]
Mumps	yes	supportive care	transmission occurs in childhood; 0% with vaccination but still endemic in parts of the world	0.5–5/100,000; reported as 1/1,000 in Japan where mumps is endemic	[67]
Neisseria meningitidis	yes	antibiotics	transmission typically occurs in childhood	23.9%	[68]
Streptoccocus pneumoniae	yes	antibiotics	transmission typically occurs in childhood	35.9%	[68]
VZV	yes	acyclovir and prednisone	transmission typically occurs in childhood	7–85%	[61]

CMV = Cytomegalovirus; HAART = highly active antiretroviral therapy; HIV = human immunodeficiency virus; HL = hearing loss; HSV = Herpes simplex virus; LCMV = lymphocytic choriomeningitis virus; NA = not applicable; ND = not described; VZV = Varicella zoster virus.

and diagnostic power of molecular genetic testing. The success of this testing is contingent on reliable understanding of genes involved in irreplaceable auditory functioning.

Since a major aim of the field is the identification and characterization of novel genes underlying disorders such as NSHL, this chapter will provide a brief summary of the current field through the lens of a modern day 'gene hunter.' Herein, we describe fundamental concepts of the genetics of NSHL that either help or hinder novel gene identification, pivotal breakthroughs that have revolutionized conventional candidate gene approaches and provide an outlook for the field.

Fundamental Concepts of Nonsyndromic Hearing Loss Genetics

Hereditary hearing loss in humans is particularly interesting because it exemplifies several principles of genetics exceedingly well that have either complicated or supported novel gene discovery.

The role of nonrandom or positive assortative mating in the genetics of deafness is well recognized. Deafness is a classic example of a trait exhibiting strong preferential selection shaping mating structures. Deaf-deaf marriages occur at a greater frequency than what would be assumed under a random mating pattern. Interestingly, a significantly large proportion of the offspring from these unions are normacusis (normal hearing), reflecting not only the diverse aetiologies that can cause hearing loss (i.e. environmental vs. genetic) but also suggesting that either recessive inheritance or weakly penetrant mutations in a variety of different genes are important for conferring hearing loss [6]. These children are more likely to know sign languages, which are heavily categorized by sociocultural language communities, and therefore more likely to shift mating structures toward selecting a partner with hearing loss. Across several generations of marriages among the deaf, it is not completely uncommon

to see two or more distinct forms of deafness segregating in a nuclear family [7]. The occurrence of multiple deafness loci in a family can complicate gene discovery using classical methods such as linkage analysis.

The resounding success in the identification of autosomal recessive nonsyndromic hearing loss (ARNSHL) genes has been largely due to the fact that many of these genes were discovered through linkage analyses or homozygosity mapping approaches in large consanguineous families (as evident in the small subset of genes shown in table 3). There are various factors influencing marriage structures around the world that have the potential of impacting consanguinity, with religion, sociocultural traditions, and geography as examples [3]. The extent of consanguineous marriage is extremely variable with high rates reported in the Middle East, South Asia and sub-Saharan Africa. For instance, a remarkable 60% of marriages in Pakistan are consanguineous, with ~80% of those between first degree cousins [8]. Offspring of such marriages theoretically inherit 6.25% of all loci identically by descent through a common ancestor, significantly increasing the likelihood of homozygous variant transmission from carrier parents [9]. Genetic studies of Pakistani kindred have uncovered over 35 NSHL genes and loci [10], reinforcing the utility certain populations can provide for candidate gene studies.

Although the degree of homozygosity in individual genomes is shaped by population history and cultural factors [11], genetic studies can also be enhanced from including certain populations not practicing consanguineous marriage but in whom founder mutations are prevalent. Studies of communities such as the Amish have been very important for new disease gene discovery in hearing loss with an example of such success evident in a founder mutation detected in the autosomal recessive gene *SLITRK6* (c.890C>A; p.S297X) in an old-order Amish family. This mutation was identified in a single family with 3 affected siblings having deafness and high myopia [12].

Table 3. Hearing loss genes identified by high-throughput sequencing approaches

DFN locus	Gene symbol	Gene name	MIM	Ethnicity	Consanguinity	Method of detection	Reference
Autosomal dominant nonsyndromic hearing loss							
DFNA4B	CEACAM16	carcinoembryonic antigen related cell adhesion molecule 16	*614591	American	no	GWL, WES	[69, 70]
DFNA41	P2RX2	purinergic receptor P2X, ligand gated ion channel 2	*600844	Chinese	no	GWL, TE and MPS	[71, 72]
DFNA56	TNC	tenascin C	*187380	Chinese	no	GWL, WES	[73]
DFNA65	TBC1D24	TBC1 domain family member 24	*613577	Chinese, American	no, no	IBD mapping and WES; GWL, WES	[74, 75]
DFNA66	CD164	CD164 molecule	*603356	Danish	no	GWL, TE and MPS	[76]
DFNA67	OSBPL2	oxysterol binding protein like 2	*606731	German	no	GWL, WES	[77]
DFNA68	HOMER2	Homer scaffolding protein 2	*604799	European descent	no	WES	[78]
	MCM2	minichromosome maintenance complex component 2	*116945	Chinese	no	WES	[79]
Autosomal recessive nonsyndromic hearing loss							
DFNB32/82	GPSM2	G-protein signaling modulator 2	*609245	Palestinian	yes	GWL, HM, WES	[42, 80]
DFNB44	ADCY1	adenylate cyclase 1	*103072	Pakistani	yes	GWL, WES	[81, 82]
DFNB49	BDP1	B double prime 1, subunit of RNA polymerase III transcription initiation factor IIIB	*607012	Qatari	yes	GWL, WES	[83]
DFNB66	DCDC2	doublecortin domain containing 2	*605755	Tunisian	yes	GWL, WES	[84, 85]
DFNB68	S1PR2	sphingosine-1-phosphate receptor 2	*605111	Pakistani	yes	GWL, WES	[86, 87]
DFNB79	TPRN	taperin	*613354	Pakistani, Moroccan	yes, yes	GWL, candidate gene sequencing; TE and MPS	[40, 41, 88]
DFNB84B	OTOGL	otogelin-like	*614925	Turkish, Dutch	yes, no	AM, GWL, WES; AM candidate gene sequencing	[89]
DFNB86	TBC1D24	TBC1 domain family member 24	*613577	Pakistani	yes	GWL, HM, WES	[90, 91]
DFNB88	ELMOD3	ELMO/CED-12 domain containing 3	*615427	Pakistani	yes	GWL, HM, WES	[92]
DFNB89	KARS	lysyl-tRNA synthetase	*601421	Pakistani	yes	GWL, HM, WES	[93, 94]
DFNB93	CABP2	calcium binding protein 2	*607314	Iranian	yes	GWL, TE and MPS	[95, 96]

Table 3. Continued

DFN locus	Gene symbol	Gene name	MIM	Ethnicity	Consanguinity	Method of detection	Reference
DFNB94	NARS2	asparaginyl-tRNA synthetase 2, mitochondrial	*612803	Pakistani	yes	GWL, WES	[97]
DFNB97	MET	MET proto-oncogene, receptor tyrosine kinase	*164860	Pakistani	yes	GWL, WES	[98]
DFNB98	TSPEAR	thrombospondin-type laminin G domain and EAR repeats	*612920	Iranian	yes	GWL, WFS	[99]
DFNB99	TMEM132E	transmembrane protein 132E	*616178	Chinese	yes	GWL, WES	[100]
DFNB101	GRXCR2	glutaredoxin, cysteine rich 2	*615762	Pakistani	yes	HM, WES	[101]
DFNB102	EPS8	epidermal growth factor receptor pathway substrate 8	*600206	Algerian	yes	WES	[102]
DFNB103	CLIC5	chloride intracellular channel 5	*607293	Turkish	yes	HM, WES	[103]
DFNB104	FAM65B	family with sequence similarity 65 member B	*611410	Turkish	yes	WES	[104]
	EPS8L2	EPS8 like 2	*614988	Algerian	yes	WES	[105]
X-linked nonsyndromic hearing loss							
DFNX4	SMPX	small muscle protein, X-linked	*300226	Dutch, Spanish, German	no	linkage and TE and MPS	[106–108]
DFNX5	AIFM1	apoptosis inducing factor, mitochondria associated 1	*300169	Chinese	no	linkage and WES	[109, 110]
DFNX6	COL4A6	collagen type IV alpha 6	*303631	Hungarian	no	linkage and WES of X chromosome	[34]

AM = Autozygosity mapping; GWL = genome-wide linkage; HM = homozygosity mapping; IBD = identity by descent; MPS = massively parallel sequencing; TE = targeted enrichment; WES = whole-exome sequencing.

Genetic studies such as those conducted in Pakistani kindred have taught us an important lesson: hearing loss demonstrates several layers of appreciable heterogeneity (i.e. genetic, allelic, and clinical), creating an additional challenge for genetic studies aiming to elucidate novel genes and establish phenotype correlations [13]. NSHL has been described as manifesting a high degree of genetic heterogeneity with estimates of up to 1% of human genes indispensable for normal hearing [14]. The growing list of genes suggests this estimate could be plausible, with nearly 100 NSHL genes already identified to date [3] (fig. 1) and many additional loci mapped through genome-wide linkage and/or homozygosity mapping but lacking an identified causative gene [15]. Multiple

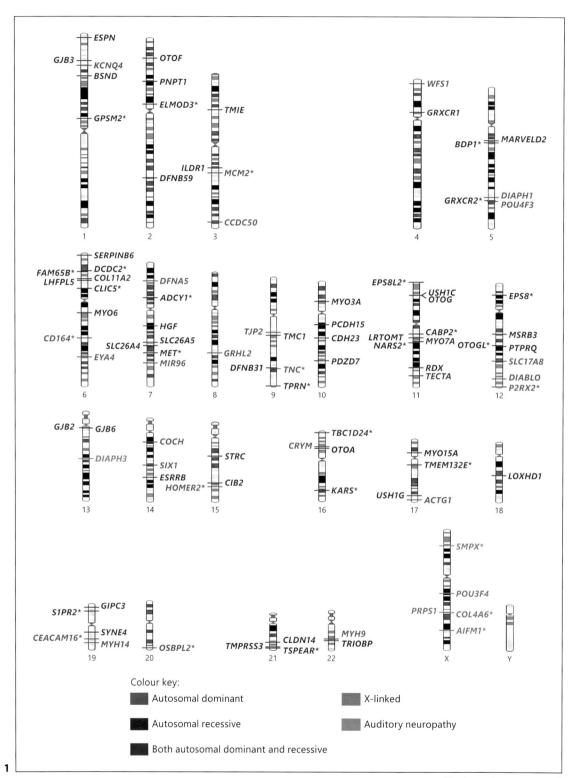

(For legend see next page.)

NSHL genes have been identified on the X chromosome and almost every autosome, highlighting a high degree of locus heterogeneity. Furthermore, as the mutation spectrum of a gene becomes apparent, it is clear that sometimes an excess of hundreds of different alleles show pleiotropic effects. For example, *MYO7A* is associated with both autosomal recessive and dominant forms of NSHL, as well as Usher syndrome types 1 and 2 as retinitis pigmentosa and vestibular dysfunction onset become clear [16]. To further complicate this clinical diversity using autosomal dominant nonsyndromic hearing loss (ADNSHL) as an example, extensive phenotypic variation has been described in affected members of a family cosegregating a mutation and among unrelated individuals with different mutations in the same gene [17]. Some of the phenotypic variation surrounding severity, progression and age of onset is thought to be due to environmental or secondary genetic factors such as variable expressivity of the disease [17]. Both allelic and clinical heterogeneity are problematic for mutation-based counselling, since genotype does not always predict phenotypic outcome. Moreover, genetic modifiers, penetrance, and digenic inheritance are also under-researched interests of the field whose results will be paramount to begin clarifying some of these observations.

The search for novel genes has consistently demonstrated a degree of unpredictability on the basis of expression data or known/putative gene function. This is especially problematic using conventional prioritized candidate gene approaches in a mapped locus, occasionally with a physical mapped distance on the scale of tens of megabases, for single gene Sanger sequencing. NSHL genes can have ubiquitous expression analogous to that of a housekeeping gene (i.e. *ACTG1*) [18, 19], or expression specific to the inner ear implicating specialized function (i.e. *TECTA*, *OTOA*, *OTOG*) [20]. NSHL genes comprise a vast diversity of gene functions, encoding a wide array of protein products with varied functions ranging from ion homeostasis to protease inhibitor activity. For example, hepatocyte growth factor encoded by *HGF* is associated with ARNSHL (DFNB39) and is important for diverse biological functions [21]. It was initially identified as a mitogen for mature cultured parenchymal hepatocytes and found to act as a hypotrophic factor triggering liver regeneration after partial hepatectomy and liver injury [22]. Furthermore, HGF is described as a motogen and as a fibroblast-secreted scatter factor mediating epithelial cell dispersion in culture [23], as a factor in erythroid differentiation [24], and as an important player in neuronal survival [25] and wound healing [26]. As part of HGF-Met signaling pathway activation, an important pathway in normal development, it has been implicated in the pathogenesis in most types of human solid tumours [27]. A consanguineous Pakistani family with ARNSHL originally mapped the DFNB39 locus to a 17.6-Mb interval on chromosome 7q [28]. Several additional families showing overlapping linkage to DFNB39 were used to reduce the linkage interval to 1.187 Mb [21]. All coding exons, as well as intra- and intergenic regions of 13 genes either inside or just outside the minimal linkage interval were directly sequenced. Homozygous changes including 2 deletions of highly conserved regulatory regions in intron 4 (c.482 + 1986_1988del and c.482 + 1991_2000del), as well as a synonymous substitution (c.495G>A; p.S165S) impacting normal splicing of exon 5 were identified in a total of 41 Indian and Pakistani

Fig. 1. Cytogenetic locations of known nonsyndromic deafness genes. Genes that were identified using high-throughput sequencing technologies are marked with an asterisk. Blue, red, violet, and orange represent genes associated with autosomal dominant, autosomal recessive, both autosomal dominant and recessive, and X-linked inheritance patterns of hearing loss. Green represents an auditory neuropathy gene. The ideogram was arranged using Ensembl GRCh38 version 78.

families. Mouse models investigating *Hgf* dysregulation result in deafness. It is thought that dysregulation of *Hgf* isoforms cause the specific cochlear pathology underlying DFNB39 deafness [21]. In summary, associating mutations in a gene such as *HGF* with particularly diverse biological function to hearing loss is not intuitive.

There is, however, one area of NSHL appearing to follow some degree of order and predictability, namely familial hearing loss. The inheritance patterns and clinical presentation of NSHL have proven a valuable starting point for understanding familial hearing loss. Although certain notable exceptions exist among the already identified genes, our current understanding suggests these incidences are relatively rare. Despite many of the basic inconsistencies that complicate correct genotype-phenotype correlations (with examples described below), their continued reporting in genes with presently very few families described will support further clinical awareness.

ARNSHL is generally sensorineural, nonprogressive and severe-to-profound across all frequencies with a congenital or prelingual onset. Considering the genetic heterogeneity defining NSHL, it is unexpected to find that a single gene, *GJB2*, resolves up to 50% of hearing loss cases in certain populations and is the most prevalent gene involved in NSHL. Mutations in *GJB2* have been reported to cause both autosomal recessive (DFNB1A) and autosomal dominant (DFNA3A) hearing loss; however, the autosomal recessive forms dominate the *GJB2* mutation spectrum. Due to the relative ease of direct sequencing of the protein-coding region of this gene, found in a single exon, it is the most logical starting point for genetic diagnostic testing, or exclusionary testing in cases not clinically fitting typical *GJB2* hearing loss.

ARNSHL generally appears in families as sporadic, without previous family history, or can be recurrent among siblings when the parents are both normacusis carriers for NSHL. Undoubted-

ly there are several exceptions to classic ARNSHL, with one example being the gene *SERPINB6* causing DFNB91. A consanguineous Turkish family with a homozygous *SERPINB6* nonsense mutation (c.733G>T; p.E245X) had reported a probable but uncertain sensorineural, postlingual onset with progressive, moderate-to-severe hearing loss that left some residual hearing in all affected family members [29].

ADNSHL almost always has a postlingual onset, sometimes with an onset after the third decade of life, and is progressive. An exception to the typical description of ADNSHL is seen in the gene *CRYM* [30]. Two pedigrees have been described with mutations in this gene, one with a de novo (c.945A>T; p.X315Y) mutation and the other with a maternally inherited (c.941A>C; p.K314T) mutation. Affected individuals showed onset between 1 and 2 years of age, and one of the 2 probands reported nonprogressive hearing loss [30]. Through the collection of multiple audiogram measurements over time, or even by virtue of assembling audiogram thresholds from members of the same family together to construct one audio-profile, the rate of hearing loss progression can be calculated as an annual threshold deterioration expressed in dB (hearing level) lost per year and can correlate a predictable or variable progressive hearing loss in a family [31]. As opposed to their recessive counterparts, autosomal dominant forms are easily identifiable in families with multiple generations affected, but can also appear sporadic with an underlying de novo mutation, as with one of the described *CRYM* pedigrees [30]. The distinction between ADNSHL and presbycusis or age-related hearing loss becomes clouded especially with deficits seen in the higher frequencies and onset later in life [17].

A disproportionate sex ratio for deafness has long been observed, in line with the observation that 4% of protein-coding genes reside on the X chromosome. Although it is thought that 1 out of every 50,000 individuals have X-linked NSHL, this may be an underestimation, as pedigree analyses in X-linked families can be misleading and appear as an autosomal recessive trait, especially when sporadic cases or small pedigrees without other obviously affected female relatives are present [32]. The most compelling clue for X-linked hearing loss is that males show a significantly earlier onset with considerably greater severity as compared to females. Hearing loss in males can occur either pre- or postlingually, with either a progressive or nonprogressive course whereas females are either normacusis or show a milder hearing loss with a later onset compared to males. The hearing loss is generally sensorineural, with the exception of mutations in the genes POU3F4 and COL4A6, in which hearing loss can be mixed or conductive and even indicate abnormal inner ear morphologies together with perilymphatic gusher that are apparent during stapes or cochlear implant surgery [33, 34].

Mutations in the mitochondrial genome have been attributed to a variety of underlying syndromic and nonsyndromic forms of hearing loss. In reference to nonsyndromic forms, hearing loss can be caused by maternally inherited, acquired, heteroplasmic and homoplasmic mitochondrial mutations, and in rare cases, mutations in mitochondria arise via a de novo mechanism. When these mutations are inherited, the mother of children with pathogenic mitochondrial variants may not always have hearing loss. Variable penetrance has been marked in commonly recognized pathogenic variants in the mitochondrial genes MT-RNR1 and MT-TS1 causing NSHL. While the precise modulators of phenotypic expression are currently unknown, a threshold hypothesis attempts to explain the remarkable clinical spectrum observed in families with mutations in these genes. This hypothesis suggests a unique combination of environmental, mitochondrial, and nuclear factors push a cell over a threshold that is responsible for such observations [35]. Furthermore, the heteroplasmic ratio of a variant has been shown to be important in phenotypic outcome [36]. The m.1555A>G mutation in MT-RNR1 predisposes aminoglycoside ototoxicity susceptibility; however, a number of reports associate deafness in individuals with the m.1555A>G mutation without aminoglycoside exposure [37]. In one such example, an Arab Israeli family with a homoplasmic m.1555A>G mutation in MT-RNR1 showed severe to profound hearing loss with onset ranging from birth to adulthood [38]. As all family members were living in the same environment and without ototoxic medication exposure, it has been suggested that a nuclear modifier of deafness is underlying these phenotypic differences. The m.7445A>G mutation in MT-TS1 has been described in 3 unrelated families with highly variable penetrance, suggesting that this mitochondrial mutation is not independently sufficient to cause hearing loss [35].

The Progressive Application of High-Throughput Sequencing Technology in Deafness Research

Novel gene identification has conventionally been mediated through positional cloning strategies. Such approaches utilize gene mapping (genome-wide linkage analysis or homozygosity mapping) to localize a chromosomal interval in a large family that is followed by candidate cloning using Sanger sequencing. A major challenge resides in gene prioritization, especially in case a large locus is linked since it is both cost and time intensive to sequence every gene in a large interval. Despite this burden, there are reports of several dozen genes undergoing Sanger sequencing before a candidate gene is identified, such as the 49 genes in the DFNB70 locus that were sequenced in order to identify the gene PNPT1 [39]. Researchers rely heavily on auditory gene expression databases in several animal models (mouse, zebrafish, Drosophila) to guide gene prioritization and expedite gene discovery. As more genes and ethnic-specific deafness-associated mutations have been identified, a common approach also included exclusionary testing for mutations in known genes before working toward the positional cloning of a novel gene. However, the number and size of the genes involved in hearing loss make comprehensive Sanger sequencing impractical. Despite careful locus mapping and gene screening, the risk of missing a causative mutation in a candidate gene can be quite high; nevertheless, there have been many successes using these approaches over the years, especially those genes published before 2010 [15].

The past 3 decades have been witness to impressive breakthroughs in the identification and elucidation of gene function across the field of genetics. Unparalleled advances in genomics and technology have rendered a human genome reference sequence together with the tools to begin decoding genetic variants in the context of an underlying unresolved genetic disease. The year 2010 marked a pivotal transition in deafness research with the emergence of the first achievements using high-throughput next-generation sequencing technologies to rapidly identify genetic mutations in novel genes. These technologies have been used to empower large-scale cost-effective screening of a variety of genes and non-coding regions that permit customizable and scalable options ranging from small gene panels and custom regions of interest to whole genomes. The first 2 publications utilized targeted enrichment (TE) and massively parallel sequencing (MPS), as well as whole-exome sequencing (WES) as part of comprehensive approaches leading to the discovery of 2 ARNSHL genes.

The first gene identified from the use of TE and MPS was *TPRN* encoding taperin [40] in the ARNSHL locus DFNB79. Genome-wide linkage of a consanguineous Pakistani family mapped DFNB79 to a 3.84-Mb interval on chromosome 9q34.3 containing 113 genes [41] that was further refined to a 2.9-Mb interval containing 108 genes. A custom TE assay of the DFNB79 locus was designed to include UTRs, protein-coding, noncoding, and intergenic regions. MPS was per-formed with the Roche 454 system that uncovered a homozygous nonsense mutation (c.1056G>A, p.W352X) in a selected proband. *TPRN* was further identified in 3 additional consanguineous Pakistani families with linkage to the DFNB79 locus, all showing homozygous frameshift mutations (c.1244delC, c.44_54dup, c.42_52del). All variants were not identified in 488–500 control chromosomes from the Pakistani population and 400 chromosomes from the Coriell HD200CAU human variation panel.

The first gene identified from the use of WES was *GPSM2* responsible for DFNB82 [42]. A consanguineous Palestinian family with ARNSHL mapped a 3.1-Mb locus containing 50 annotated genes and 1 miRNA. Paired-end sequences were generated on an Illumina Genome Analyzer IIx. WES and analysis of the DFNB82 locus in a proband disclosed 73 polymorphic substitutions and 7 novel unclassified variants, two of which introduced a change in the coding amino acid. Population-matched screening of 192 hearing controls and 192 unrelated probands for the 2 amino acid altering mutations ensued with a homozygous nonsense mutation (c.875C>T; p.R127X) in the gene *GPSM2* appearing as a private mutation in the affected family.

High-throughput sequencing approaches have already shown impressive results with 31 NSHL genes identified to date employing these cutting-edge technologies (table 3), with new genes being reported frequently. The rapid pace of new gene discovery is a testament to conceptual changes in candidate approaches. In particular, many smaller families without a chance of providing informative gene mapping results can finally be included in research studies. Their utility has also shown significance in deciphering the mutational spectrum in genes with a limited number of families identified thus far.

These advanced technologies are not limited to genomic DNA applications. High-throughput transcriptomics is a highly dynamic area elucidating expression profiles in tissues of interest. The application of gene expression profiling in inner ear cells has been studied since 2002 in the rat [43] and mouse [44] using DNA microarray technology. RNA sequencing (RNA-Seq) gene profiling overcomes some of the limitations of DNA array profiling technologies. Databases such as SHIELD (Shared Harvard Inner-Ear Laboratory Database) [45] provide an extensive quantitative transcriptome catalog of fluorescence-activated cell-sorted mouse vestibular and cochlear hair cells at 4 developmental stages. For the first time, a comprehensive expression catalog of the human inner ear has been published using an RNA-Seq approach [46]. These data provide pioneering insight to the transcriptional landscape of genes in the inner ear and will serve as valuable repositories for the research community.

Bearing in mind the pace in which MPS technologies have emerged and that these technologies are still in their infancy, it is not surprising that there are still a number of limitations requiring further development. One chronic bottleneck involves engaging effective data analysis strategies in a time when genetic variant interpretation is clouded by ambiguity and understanding of the human genome changes (nearly) on a daily basis. Falsely annotated variants that are deposited in large pathogenic databases on which researchers and clinicians are reliant pose a major challenge and is evidently a systemic issue for all of human genetics. Studies aiming to detect pathogenic genetic changes in a patient group can easily fall into common pitfalls such as analyzing small cohorts, undergoing limited validation and not analyzing control populations for variant frequency [47]. One of the largest mutation repositories is the Human Gene Mutation Database (HGMD) [48] in which curators continuously re-examine the literature for updated evidence for or against pathogenic implication. A study from 2013 calculated 8.5% of HGMD variants to be present in 1,092 presumably asymptomatic control individuals from the 1000 Genomes Project (Phase 1, Version 3), with each individual having an average of 942 heterozygous and 294 homozygous variants overlapping with HGMD entries [47]. This observation reiterates the importance of careful variant assignment and for penetrance and predictive-disease considerations in presumably asymptomatic individuals. Second to this, a study evaluated false positives when analyzing 66 NSHL genes in 8,595 normal hearing controls from 12 different population groups [49]. In these 66 genes, 2,197 variants were reported as pathogenic in HGMD, dbSNP [50] and/or ClinVar [51] with 1,872 novel and 325 pathogenic variants in controls. Based on minor allele frequency threshold cut-offs, 93 pathogenic classified variants were re-categorized as benign. These data are publicly available on the Deafness Variation Database and intend to serve as a resource to aid with the interpretation of variants in NSHL [49].

In extreme cases a greater understanding of the mutational spectrum has resulted in disease gene disqualification when evidence such as healthy individuals detected with truncating mutations or high frequencies of likely deleterious mutations present in public datasets become clear. Gene disqualification has already been in discussion in the NSHL literature with discordant cosegregation observed with *MYO1A* variants [52] that even included a homozygous nonsense mutation, strongly suggesting that *MYO1A* is not required for hearing. Furthermore, in silico pathogenicity prediction tools can also be employed to support implication of variant pathogenicity, but should be used with caution, as hundreds to thousands of coding variants will be predicted as having a potentially damaging or deleterious outcome [53]. Each of the many publicly available pathogenicity prediction programs utilize different computational algorithms, running the risk of producing significantly different outcomes when analyzing even a single variant [54].

TE of a defined locus or subset of the genome, as with small deafness gene panels, restricts analysis to a manageable subset of targets of interest.

Compared to large-scale datasets such as those expected for whole genomes and whole exomes, data storage infrastructure is simplified and analysis times are greatly reduced. However, custom panels run a risk of becoming quickly out of date as new genes are discovered and require validation with every update. One alternative to small custom panels are commercially available clinical exomes such as the Kingsmore panel with 1,222 genes (version 2) or the TruSight One sequencing panel (Illumina) with 4,813 genes that already include many of the known deafness genes. One advantage to using these panels is that sequencing data from other poorly characterized genes (especially in the case of the TruSight One panel) are available that permit a rapid expansion of analysis in a research context to include these genes after exclusionary testing of known genes yields an uninformative result. One drawback is that not all hearing loss genes are already included and the risk of detecting unintended incidental findings or secondary variants is high. Furthermore, commercially available library preparation enrichment kits are generally unlikely to include all protein-encoding exons and will miss potentially relevant deep intronic and promoter variants. Pseudogenes, repetitive elements and promoters are also likely to undergo capture difficulties. The short reads that are typical for currently used MPS systems are also problematic for alignment of some of these harder-to-sequence regions, as well as detecting structural variation in repetitive sequences.

One area likely to engage bioethicists in the long term are ethical concerns raised from MPS datasets. It is usually not a question of whether clinically significant unintended findings secondary to the research aims will be generated, but how many of such findings will be detected and how these should be managed [55]. Handling of unintended incidental or secondary variants is something that will require policies defining consensus criteria, clear communication between genetic counsellors, clinicians, and patients, as well

as explicit informed consent procedures. Genomic privacy, data access rights, and the potential for discrimination are also issues for concern.

Outlook

The resonating optimism of molecular genetic diagnostic capabilities through the use of high-throughput technologies is so impressive that it is being heralded as 'the new standard of patient care' [56]. These approaches should be considered in patients without a diagnosis following single gene testing or when it provides a faster and cheaper means for accurate genetic diagnosis. In a clinical setting, considerable caution should be exercised with the assessment of gene-disease causality when returning results to patients. Guidelines are gradually emerging that will be critical for understanding the broader impact of returning poorly supported results [57]. Only after proper attention is given to clinical validity can a personalized approach to hearing loss management become possible with substantiated 'cause and effect' relationships of genetic mutations. For example, a study concluded that children with variants in *DFNB59* and *PCDH15* have poor cochlear implant performance and indistinguishable preoperative audiological and diagnostic imaging results when compared to other cochlear implant recipients with good outcomes [58]. This association is among the first to link a negative cochlear implant outcome to specific genes in absence of other clinical clues.

Notwithstanding current limitations, there is still much enthusiasm surrounding present and future developments in high-throughput sequencing that has delivered remarkable tools for researchers and diagnosticians alike. A collection of 20 independent studies using these approaches have already reported a combined diagnostic rate of 41% in hearing loss patients [56]. These cutting-edge technologies have enabled previously unimaginable testing to become a reality and are the first step toward patient-tailored therapies.

References

1 Keats BJ, Berlin CI: Genomics and hearing impairment. Genome Res 1999;9: 7–16.

2 Morton CC, Nance WE: Newborn hearing screening – a silent revolution. N Engl J Med 2006;354:2151–2164.

3 Smith RJ, Bale JF Jr, White KR: Sensorineural hearing loss in children. Lancet 2005;365:879–890.

4 Roizen NJ: Nongenetic causes of hearing loss. Ment Retard Dev Disabil Res Rev 2003;9:120–127.

5 Parker M, Bitner-Glindzicz M: Genetic investigations in childhood deafness. Arch Dis Child 2015;100:271–278.

6 Morton CC: Genetics, genomics and gene discovery in the auditory system. Hum Mol Genet 2002;11:1229–1240.

7 Nance WE, Kearsey MJ: Relevance of connexin deafness (DFNB1) to human evolution. Am J Hum Genet 2004;74: 1081–1087.

8 Hussain R, Bittles AH: The prevalence and demographic characteristics of consanguineous marriages in Pakistan. J Biosoc Sci 1998;30:261–275.

9 Woods CG, Cox J, Springell K, Hampshire DJ, Mohamed MD, et al: Quantification of homozygosity in consanguineous individuals with autosomal recessive disease. Am J Hum Genet 2006;78:889–896.

10 Van Camp G, Smith RJH: Hereditary Hearing Loss Homepage. Updated May 13, 2015. http://hereditaryhearingloss. org.

11 Pemberton TJ, Absher D, Feldman MW, Myers RM, Rosenberg NA, Li JZ: Genomic patterns of homozygosity in worldwide human populations. Am J Hum Genet 2012;91:275–292.

12 Tekin M, Chioza BA, Matsumoto Y, Diaz-Horta O, Cross HE, et al: SLITRK6 mutations cause myopia and deafness in humans and mice. J Clin Invest 2013; 123:2094–2102.

13 Petersen MB, Willems PJ: Non-syndromic, autosomal-recessive deafness. Clin Genet 2006;69:371–392.

14 Friedman TB, Griffith AJ: Human nonsyndromic sensorineural deafness. Annu Rev Genomics Hum Genet 2003;4: 341–402.

15 Vona B, Nanda I, Hofrichter MA, Shehata-Dieler W, Haaf T: Non-syndromic hearing loss gene identification: a brief history and glimpse into the future. Mol Cell Probes 2015;29:260–270.

16 Rong W, Chen X, Zhao K, Liu Y, Liu X, et al: Novel and recurrent MYO7A mutations in Usher syndrome type 1 and type 2. PLoS One 2014;9:e97808.

17 Greene CC, McMillan PM, Barker SE, Kurnool P, Lomax MI, et al: DFNA25, a novel locus for dominant nonsyndromic hereditary hearing impairment, maps to 12q21–24. Am J Hum Genet 2001;68: 254–260.

18 van Wijk E, Krieger E, Kemperman MH, De Leenheer EM, Huygen PL, et al: A mutation in the gamma actin 1 (ACTG1) gene causes autosomal dominant hearing loss (DFNA20/26). J Med Genet 2003;40:879–884.

19 Zhu M, Yang T, Wei S, DeWan AT, Morell RJ, et al: Mutations in the gamma-actin gene (ACTG1) are associated with dominant progressive deafness (DFNA20/26). Am J Hum Genet 2003; 73:1082–1091.

20 Zwaenepoel I, Mustapha M, Leibovici M, Verpy E, Goodyear R, et al: Otoancorin, an inner ear protein restricted to the interface between the apical surface of sensory epithelia and their overlying acellular gels, is defective in autosomal recessive deafness DFNB22. Proc Natl Acad Sci U S A 2002;99:6240–6245.

21 Schultz JM, Khan SN, Ahmed ZM, Riazuddin S, Waryah AM, et al: Noncoding mutations of HGF are associated with nonsyndromic hearing loss, DFNB39. Am J Hum Genet 2009;85: 25–39.

22 Nakamura T, Nishizawa T, Hagiya M, Seki T, Shimonishi M, et al: Molecular cloning and expression of human hepatocyte growth factor. Nature 1989;342: 440–443.

23 Stoker M, Gherardi E, Perryman M, Gray J: Scatter factor is a fibroblast-derived modulator of epithelial cell mobility. Nature 1987;327:239–242.

24 Kmiecik TE, Keller JR, Rosen E, Vande Woude GF: Hepatocyte growth factor is a synergistic factor for the growth of hematopoietic progenitor cells. Blood 1992;80:2454–2457.

25 Hayashi K, Morishita R, Nakagami H, Yoshimura S, Hara A, et al: Gene therapy for preventing neuronal death using hepatocyte growth factor: in vivo gene transfer of HGF to subarachnoid space prevents delayed neuronal death in gerbil hippocampal CA1 neurons. Gene Ther 2001;8:1167–1173.

26 Bevan D, Gherardi E, Fan TP, Edwards D, Warn R: Diverse and potent activities of HGF/SF in skin wound repair. J Pathol 2004;203:831–838.

27 Zhang YW, Vande Woude GF: HGF/SF-met signaling in the control of branching morphogenesis and invasion. J Cell Biochem 2003;88:408–417.

28 Wajid M, Abbasi AA, Ansar M, Pham TL, Yan K, et al: DFNB39, a recessive form of sensorineural hearing impairment, maps to chromosome 7q11.22–q21.12. Eur J Hum Genet 2003;11:812–815.

29 Sirmaci A, Erbek S, Price J, Huang M, Duman D, et al: A truncating mutation in SERPINB6 is associated with autosomal-recessive nonsyndromic sensorineural hearing loss. Am J Hum Genet 2010;86:797–804.

30 Abe S, Katagiri T, Saito-Hisaminato A, Usami S, Inoue Y, et al: Identification of CRYM as a candidate responsible for nonsyndromic deafness, through cDNA microarray analysis of human cochlear and vestibular tissues. Am J Hum Genet 2003;72:73–82.

31 Vona B, Nanda I, Neuner C, Müller T, Haaf T: Confirmation of GRHL2 as the gene for the DFNA28 locus. Am J Med Genet A 2013;161A:2060–2065.

32 Petersen MB, Wang Q, Willems PJ: Sex-linked deafness. Clin Genet 2008;73: 14–23.

33 de Kok YJ, van der Maarel SM, Bitner-Glindzicz M, Huber I, Monaco AP, et al: Association between X-linked mixed deafness and mutations in the POU domain gene POU3F4. Science 1995;267: 685–688.

34 Rost S, Bach E, Neuner C, Nanda I, Dysek S, et al: Novel form of X-linked nonsyndromic hearing loss with cochlear malformation caused by a mutation in the type IV collagen gene COL4A6. Eur J Hum Genet 2014;22:208–215.

35 Fischel-Ghodsian N: Mitochondrial mutations and hearing loss: paradigm for mitochondrial genetics. Am J Hum Genet 1998;62:15–19.

36 del Castillo FJ, Rodríguez-Ballesteros M, Martín Y, Arellano B, Gallo-Terán J, et al: Heteroplasmy for the 1555A>G mutation in the mitochondrial 12S rRNA gene in six Spanish families with nonsyndromic hearing loss. J Med Genet 2003;40:632–636.

37 el-Schahawi M, López de Munain A, Sarrazin AM, Shanske AL, Basirico M, et al: Two large Spanish pedigrees with nonsyndromic sensorineural deafness and the mtDNA mutation at nt 1555 in the 12S rRNA gene: evidence of heteroplasmy. Neurology 1997;48:453–456.

38 Jaber L, Shohat M, Bu X, Fischel-Ghodsian N, Yang HY, et al: Sensorineural deafness inherited as a tissue specific mitochondrial disorder. J Med Genet 1992;29:86–90.

39 von Ameln S, Wang G, Boulouiz R, Rutherford MA, Smith GM, et al: A mutation in PNPT1, encoding mitochondrial-RNA-import protein PNPase, causes hereditary hearing loss. Am J Hum Genet 2012;91:919–927.

40 Rehman AU, Morell RJ, Belyantseva IA, Khan SY, Boger ET, et al: Targeted capture and next-generation sequencing identifies C9orf75, encoding taperin, as the mutated gene in nonsyndromic deafness DFNB79. Am J Hum Genet 2010;86:378–388.

41 Khan SY, Riazuddin S, Shahzad M, Ahmed N, Zafar AU, et al: DFNB79: reincarnation of a nonsyndromic deafness locus on chromosome 9q34.3. Eur J Hum Genet 2010;18:125–129.

42 Walsh T, Shahin H, Elkan-Miller T, Lee MK, Thornton AM, et al: Whole exome sequencing and homozygosity mapping identify mutation in the cell polarity protein GPSM2 as the cause of nonsyndromic hearing loss DFNB82. Am J Hum Genet 2010;87:90–94.

43 Cho Y, Gong TW, Stover T, Lomax MI, Altschuler RA: Gene expression profiles of the rat cochlea, cochlear nucleus, and inferior colliculus. J Assoc Res Otolaryngol 2002;3:54–67.

44 Chen ZY, Corey DP: An inner ear gene expression database. J Assoc Res Otolaryngol 2002;3:140–148.

45 Scheffer DI, Shen J, Corey DP, Chen ZY: Gene expression by mouse inner ear hair cells during development. J Neurosci 2015;35:6366–6380.

46 Schrauwen I, Hasin-Brumshtein Y, Corneveaux JJ, Ohmen J, White C, et al: A comprehensive catalogue of the coding and non-coding transcripts of the human inner ear. Hear Res 2015; E-pub ahead of print.

47 Cassa CA, Tong MY, Jordan DM: Large numbers of genetic variants considered to be pathogenic are common in asymptomatic individuals. Hum Mutat 2013; 34:1216–1220.

48 Stenson PD, Mort M, Ball EV, Shaw K, Phillips A, Cooper DN: The Human Gene Mutation Database: building a comprehensive mutation repository for clinical and molecular genetics, diagnostic testing and personalized genomic medicine. Hum Genet 2014;133:1–9.

49 Shearer AE, Eppsteiner RW, Booth KT, Ephraim SS, Gurrola J 2nd, et al: Utilizing ethnic-specific differences in minor allele frequency to recategorize reported pathogenic deafness variants. Am J Hum Genet 2014;95:445–453.

50 Sherry ST, Ward MH, Kholodov M, Baker J, Phan L, et al: dbSNP: the NCBI database of genetic variation. Nucleic Acids Res 2001;29:308–311.

51 Landrum MJ, Lee JM, Benson M, Brown G, Chao C, et al: ClinVar: public archive of interpretations of clinically relevant variants. Nucleic Acids Res 2016; 44:D862–D868.

52 Eisenberger T, Di Donato N, Baig SM, Neuhaus C, Beyer A, et al: Targeted and genomewide NGS data disqualify mutations in MYO1A, the 'DFNA48 gene', as a cause of deafness. Hum Mutat 2014; 35:565–570.

53 MacArthur DG, Manolio TA, Dimmock DP, Rehm HL, Shendure J, et al: Guidelines for investigating causality of sequence variants in human disease. Nature 2014;508:469–476.

54 Walters-Sen LC, Hashimoto S, Thrush DL, Reshmi S, Gastier-Foster JM, et al: Variability in pathogenicity prediction programs: impact on clinical diagnostics. Mol Genet Genomic Med 2015;3: 99–110.

55 Abdul-Karim R, Berkman BE, Wendler D, Rid A, Khan J, et al: Disclosure of incidental findings from next-generation sequencing in pediatric genomic research. Pediatrics 2013;131:564–571.

56 Shearer AE, Smith RJ: Massively parallel sequencing for genetic diagnosis of hearing loss: the new standard of care. Otolaryngol Head Neck Surg 2015;153: 175–182.

57 Abou Tayoun AN, Al Turki SH, Oza AM, Bowser MJ, Hernandez AL, et al: Improving hearing loss gene testing: a systematic review of gene evidence toward more efficient next-generation sequencing-based diagnostic testing and interpretation. Genet Med 2015; E-pub ahead of print.

58 Wu CC, Lin YH, Liu TC, Lin KN, Yang WS, et al: Identifying children with poor cochlear implantation outcomes using massively parallel sequencing. Medicine (Baltimore) 2015;94:e1073.

59 Hoefsloot LH, Feenstra I, Kunst HP, Kremer H: Genotype phenotype correlations for hearing impairment: approaches to management. Clin Genet 2014;85: 514–523.

60 Kimberlin DW, Jester PM, Sanchez PJ, Ahmed A, Arav-Boger R, et al: Valganciclovir for symptomatic congenital cytomegalovirus disease. N Engl J Med 2015; 372:933–943.

61 Cohen BE, Durstenfeld A, Roehm PC: Viral causes of hearing loss: a review for hearing health professionals. Trends Hear 2014;18:1–17.

62 Salviz M, Montoya JG, Nadol JB, Santos F: Otopathology in congenital toxoplasmosis. Otol Neurotol 2013;34:1165–1169.

63 Montoya JG, Liesenfeld O: Toxoplasmosis. Lancet 2004;363:1965–1976.

64 al Muhaimeed H, Zakzouk SM: Hearing loss and herpes simplex. J Trop Pediatr 1997;43:20–24.

65 Espiney Amaro C, Montalvao P, Huins C, Saraiva J: Lyme disease: sudden hearing loss as the sole presentation. J Laryngol Otol 2015;129:183–186.

66 Edmond K, Clark A, Korczak VS, Sanderson C, Griffiths UK, Rudan I: Global and regional risk of disabling sequelae from bacterial meningitis: a systematic review and meta-analysis. Lancet Infect Dis 2010;10:317–328.

67 Hashimoto H, Fujioka M, Kinumaki H; Kinki Ambulatory Pediatrics Study Group: An office-based prospective study of deafness in mumps. Pediatr Infect Dis J 2009;28:173–175.

68 Kutz JW, Simon LM, Chennupati SK, Giannoni CM, Manolidis S: Clinical predictors for hearing loss in children with bacterial meningitis. Arch Otolaryngol Head Neck Surg 2006;132:941–945.

69 Zheng J, Miller KK, Yang T, Hildebrand MS, Shearer AE, et al: Carcinoembryonic antigen-related cell adhesion molecule 16 interacts with alpha-tectorin and is mutated in autosomal dominant hearing loss (DFNA4). Proc Natl Acad Sci U S A 2011;108:4218–4223.

70 Chen AH, Ni L, Fukushima K, Marietta J, O'Neill M, et al: Linkage of a gene for dominant non-syndromic deafness to chromosome 19. Hum Mol Genet 1995; 4:1073–1076.

71 Yan D, Zhu Y, Walsh T, Xie D, Yuan H, et al: Mutation of the ATP-gated P2X(2) receptor leads to progressive hearing loss and increased susceptibility to noise. Proc Natl Acad Sci U S A 2013; 110:2228–2233.

72 Blanton SH, Liang CY, Cai MW, Pandya A, Du LL, et al: A novel locus for autosomal dominant non-syndromic deafness (DFNA41) maps to chromosome 12q24-qter. J Med Genet 2002;39:567–570.

73 Zhao Y, Zhao F, Zong L, Zhang P, Guan L, et al: Exome sequencing and linkage analysis identified tenascin-C *(TNC)* as a novel causative gene in nonsyndromic hearing loss. PLoS One 2013;8:e69549.

74 Azaiez H, Booth KT, Bu F, Huygen P, Shibata SB, et al: *TBC1D24* mutation causes autosomal dominant non-syndromic hearing loss. Hum Mutat 2014; 35:819–823.

75 Zhang L, Hu L, Chai Y, Pang X, Yang T, Wu H: A dominant mutation in the stereocilia-expressing gene *TBC1D24* is a probable cause for nonsyndromic hearing impairment. Hum Mutat 2014;35: 814–818.

76 Nyegaard M, Rendtorff ND, Nielsen MS, Corydon TJ, Demontis D, et al: A novel locus harbouring a functional *CD164* nonsense mutation identified in a large Danish family with nonsyndromic hearing impairment. PLoS Genet 2015; 11:e1005386.

77 Thoenes M, Zimmermann U, Ebermann I, Ptok M, Lewis MA, et al: *OSBPL2* encodes a protein of inner and outer hair cell stereocilia and is mutated in autosomal dominant hearing loss (DFNA67). Orphanet J Rare Dis 2015; 10:15.

78 Azaiez H, Decker AR, Booth KT, Simpson AC, Shearer AE, et al: HOMER2, a stereociliary scaffolding protein, is essential for normal hearing in humans and mice. PLoS Genet 2015; 11:e1005137.

79 Gao J, Wang Q, Dong C, Chen S, Qi Y, Liu Y: Whole exome sequencing identified *MCM2* as a novel causative gene for autosomal dominant nonsyndromic deafness in a Chinese family. PLoS One 2015;10:e0133522.

80 Masmoudi S, Tlili A, Majava M, Ghorbel AM, Chardenoux S, et al: Mapping of a new autosomal recessive nonsyndromic hearing loss locus (DFNB32) to chromosome 1p13.3–22.1. Eur J Hum Genet 2003;11:185–188.

81 Santos-Cortez RL, Lee K, Giese AP, Ansar M, Amin-Ud-Din M, et al: Adenylate cyclase 1 *(ADCY1)* mutations cause recessive hearing impairment in humans and defects in hair cell function and hearing in zebrafish. Hum Mol Genet 2014;23:3289–3298.

82 Ansar M, Chahrour MH, Amin Ud Din M, Arshad M, Haque S, et al: DFNB44, a novel autosomal recessive non-syndromic hearing impairment locus, maps to chromosome 7p14.1–q11.22. Hum Hered 2004;57:195–199.

83 Girotto G, Abdulhadi K, Buniello A, Vozzi D, Licastro D, et al: Linkage study and exome sequencing identify a *BDP1* mutation associated with hereditary hearing loss. PLoS One 2013;8:e80323.

84 Grati M, Chakchouk I, Ma Q, Bensaid M, Desmidt A, et al: A missense mutation in *DCDC2* causes human recessive deafness DFNB66, likely by interfering with sensory hair cell and supporting cell cilia length regulation. Hum Mol Genet 2015;24:2482–2491.

85 Tlili A, Männikkö M, Charfedine I, Lahmar I, Benzina Z, et al: A novel autosomal recessive non-syndromic deafness locus, DFNB66, maps to chromosome 6p21.2–22.3 in a large Tunisian consanguineous family. Hum Hered 2005;60: 123–128.

86 Santos RL, Hassan MJ, Sikandar S, Lee K, Ali G, et al: DFNB68, a novel autosomal recessive non-syndromic hearing impairment locus at chromosomal region 19p13.2. Hum Genet 2006;120: 85–92.

87 Santos-Cortez RL, Faridi R, Rehman AU, Lee K, Ansar M, et al: Autosomal-recessive hearing impairment due to rare missense variants within *S1PR2*. Am J Hum Genet 2016;98:331–338.

88 Li Y, Pohl E, Boulouiz R, Schraders M, Nürnberg G, et al: Mutations in *TPRN* cause a progressive form of autosomal-recessive nonsyndromic hearing loss. Am J Hum Genet 2010;86:479–484.

89 Yariz KO, Duman D, Seco CZ, Dallman J, Huang M, et al: Mutations in *OTOGL*, encoding the inner ear protein otogelin-like, cause moderate sensorineural hearing loss. Am J Hum Genet 2012;91:872–882.

90 Rehman AU, Santos-Cortez RL, Morell RJ, Drummond MC, Ito T, et al: Mutations in *TBC1D24*, a gene associated with epilepsy, also cause nonsyndromic deafness DFNB86. Am J Hum Genet 2014;94:144–152.

91 Ali RA, Rehman AU, Khan SN, Husnain T, Riazuddin S, et al: DFNB86, a novel autosomal recessive non-syndromic deafness locus on chromosome 16p13.3. Clin Genet 2012;81:498–500.

92 Jaworek TJ, Richard EM, Ivanova AA, Giese AP, Choo DI, et al: An alteration in ELMOD3, an Arl2 GTPase-activating protein, is associated with hearing impairment in humans. PLoS Genet 2013; 9:e1003774.

93 Santos-Cortez RL, Lee K, Azeem Z, Antonellis PJ, Pollock LM, et al: Mutations in *KARS*, encoding lysyl-tRNA synthetase, cause autosomal-recessive nonsyndromic hearing impairment DFNB89. Am J Hum Genet 2013;93:132–140.

94 Basit S, Lee K, Habib R, Chen L, Umm-e-Kalsoom, et al: DFNB89, a novel autosomal recessive nonsyndromic hearing impairment locus on chromosome 16q21–q23.2. Hum Genet 2011;129: 379–385.

95 Schrauwen I, Helfmann S, Inagaki A, Predoehl F, Tabatabaiefar MA, et al: A mutation in *CABP2*, expressed in cochlear hair cells, causes autosomal-recessive hearing impairment. Am J Hum Genet 2012;91:636–645.

96 Tabatabaiefar MA, Alasti F, Shariati L, Farrokhi E, Fransen E, et al: DFNB93, a novel locus for autosomal recessive moderate-to-severe hearing impairment. Clin Genet 2011;79:594–598.

97 Simon M, Richard EM, Wang X, Shahzad M, Huang VH, et al: Mutations of human *NARS2*, encoding the mitochondrial asparaginyl-tRNA synthetase, cause nonsyndromic deafness and Leigh syndrome. PLoS Genet 2015; 11:e1005097.

98 Mujtaba G, Schultz JM, Imtiaz A, Morell RJ, Friedman TB, Naz S: A mutation of *MET*, encoding hepatocyte growth factor receptor, is associated with human DFNB97 hearing loss. J Med Genet 2015; 52:548–552.

99 Delmaghani S, Aghaie A, Michalski N, Bonnet C, Weil D, Petit C: Defect in the gene encoding the EAR/EPTP domain-containing protein TSPEAR causes DFNB98 profound deafness. Hum Mol Genet 2012;21:3835–3844.

100 Li J, Zhao X, Xin Q, Shan S, Jiang B, et al: Whole-exome sequencing identifies a variant in *TMEM132E* causing autosomal-recessive nonsyndromic hearing loss DFNB99. Hum Mutat 2015;36:98–105.

101 Imtiaz A, Kohrman DC, Naz S: A frameshift mutation in *GRXCR2* causes recessively inherited hearing loss. Hum Mutat 2014;35:618–624.

102 Behlouli A, Bonnet C, Abdi S, Bouaita A, Lelli A, et al: *EPS8*, encoding an actin-binding protein of cochlear hair cell stereocilia, is a new causal gene for autosomal recessive profound deafness. Orphanet J Rare Dis 2014;9:55.

103 Seco CZ, Oonk AM, Domínguez-Ruiz M, Draaisma JM, Gandía M, et al: Progressive hearing loss and vestibular dysfunction caused by a homozygous nonsense mutation in *CLIC5*. Eur J Hum Genet 2015;23:189–194.

104 Diaz-Horta O, Subasioglu-Uzak A, Grati M, DeSmidt A, Foster J 2nd, et al: FAM65B is a membrane-associated protein of hair cell stereocilia required for hearing. Proc Natl Acad Sci U S A 2014;111:9864–9868.

105 Dahmani M, Ammar-Khodja F, Bonnet C, Lefevre GM, Hardelin JP, et al: *EPS8L2* is a new causal gene for childhood onset autosomal recessive progressive hearing loss. Orphanet J Rare Dis 2015;10:96.

106 Huebner AK, Gandia M, Frommolt P, Maak A, Wicklein EM, et al: Nonsense mutations in *SMPX*, encoding a protein responsive to physical force, result in X-chromosomal hearing loss. Am J Hum Genet 2011;88:621–627.

107 Schraders M, Haas SA, Weegerink NJ, Oostrik J, Hu H, et al: Next-generation sequencing identifies mutations of *SMPX*, which encodes the small muscle protein, X-linked, as a cause of progressive hearing impairment. Am J Hum Genet 2011;88:628–634.

108 del Castillo I, Villamar M, Sarduy M, Romero L, Herraiz C, et al: A novel locus for non-syndromic sensorineural deafness (DFN6) maps to chromosome Xp22. Hum Mol Genet 1996;5:1383–1387.

109 Wang QJ, Li QZ, Rao SQ, Lee K, Huang XS, et al: AUNX1, a novel locus responsible for X linked recessive auditory and peripheral neuropathy, maps to Xq23–27.3. J Med Genet 2006;43:e33.

110 Zong L, Guan J, Ealy M, Zhang Q, Wang D, et al: Mutations in apoptosis-inducing factor cause X-linked recessive auditory neuropathy spectrum disorder. J Med Genet 2015;52:523–531.

Thomas Haaf, MD
Institute of Human Genetics, Biocentre
Julius-Maximilians-University
Am Hubland, DE–97074 Würzburg (Germany)
E-Mail thomas.haaf@uni-wuerzburg.de

Vona B, Haaf T (eds): Genetics of Deafness. Monogr Hum Genet. Basel, Karger, 2016, vol 20, pp 73–83
(DOI: 10.1159/000444566)

Genetic Modifiers of Hearing Loss

Rizwan Yousaf[a] · Thomas B. Friedman[b] · Saima Riazuddin[a]

[a]Department of Otorhinolaryngology – Head and Neck Surgery, School of Medicine, University of Maryland, Baltimore, Md., and
[b]Laboratory of Molecular Genetics, National Institute on Deafness and Other Communication Disorders, National Institutes of
Health, Bethesda, Md., USA

Abstract

Hearing loss is a common neurosensory disorder. Mutations of many genes are associated with hearing loss, and there are a great variety of reasons for phenotypic variability, including environmental causes such as loud noise and exposure to ototoxic drugs. Additionally, there are genetic modifiers that can play a pivotal role in modulating the severity and/or the rate of hearing loss. In vertebrates including humans, genetic modifiers have been identified that affect hearing ability. Further characterization of these enhancers and suppressors of mutated genes associated with profound deafness should provide new insights into the complex molecular and functional networks essential for sound transduction and might reveal novel targets for potential therapeutic interventions to circumvent hearing loss.   © 2016 S. Karger AG, Basel

Hearing Loss

Hearing loss is defined as a partial or complete inability to perceive sound, and is a common communication disorder. Approximately 360 million people worldwide have a hearing loss, of which 328 million are adults [1]. In many countries, detection of a hearing loss may occur during new-born hearing screening, or the onset may be delayed until later in life. On an average, 1 in every 500 newborns has congenital hearing loss; the rate increases during adolescence to 3.5 per 1,000 [2]. One-third of people older than 65 years experience an age-related hearing loss [1]. A genetic etiology of congenital hearing loss accounts for ~70% of these cases, whereas nongenetic factors contribute to the remaining 30% [2]. Nongenetic factors associated with hearing loss include environmental insults, infection, acoustic trauma, or ototoxic drugs [3–5].

Genetic forms of hearing loss can be either syndromic or nonsyndromic, depending on the phenotypic presentation. There are over 400 different genetic syndromes that have been identified with hearing loss as one of the clinical features [6] as compared to the more common nonsyndromic deafness, also referred to as isolated hearing loss. Hearing loss is a genetically and clinically heterogeneous disorder, a testament to the large number of genes required for normal functioning of the auditory system. These genes encode regulatory noncoding RNAs and a diversity of proteins responsible for the development of the auditory system, as well as, for example, fluid homeostasis and long-term maintenance of hair cells, which normally do not regenerate in mammals [7–9].

Hearing ability is also influenced by viral and bacterial infections, diet, drug ototoxicity, and exposure to damaging noise [10–13]. Mutations of different genes (genetic heterogeneity) and variants of the same gene (alleles) can also result in distinct phenotypic differences in the severity or age of onset of a hearing loss. Additionally, there may be differences in the genetic background in which modifier variants modulate the phenotypic outcome of a major mutant allele. This chapter summarizes the current knowledge about genetic modifiers of hearing loss.

Genetic Modifiers

Genetic modifiers were first documented more than a century ago when researchers observed that some traits do not follow the normal segregation ratios of a simple Mendelian trait and show an 'inconsistent inheritance' [14, 15]. In these instances, genetic elements modulate the phenotype of a mutant allele, resulting in incomplete penetrance and variable expression of an otherwise simple monogenic disorder [16–19]. Modifier alleles can exert their effects by worsening or reducing the phenotype or by suppressing the disease phenotype altogether so that it is indistinguishable from the normal range [20]. Modifiers can also affect the age of disease onset or the rate of disease progression [17, 21]. Genetic modifiers can modulate the phenotype of the mutant allele at the molecular, cellular or organ level, thus impacting the organism as a whole. A modifier may interact physically with a mutant protein or with other proteins in a pathway, which may influence the expression, function or stability of a mutant protein. Phenotypic modification can also result from the expression of one gene altering the expression of another gene [17]. One such example is observed in retinitis pigmentosa type 11, which is caused by mutations in the pre-mRNA processing factor 31 gene (PRPF31) [22]. The variability in penetrance has been attributed to the level of wild-type PRPF31 mRNA expression in these patients [23]. However, the penetrance is further reduced by transcriptional repression mediated by the CCR4-NOT transcription complex, subunit 3 gene (CNOT3) [24].

Modifiers of Hearing Loss in Mice

A modifying genetic background may result from a single dominant variant or multiple variants that together modulate the hearing phenotype [25]. Genetic modifiers can originate as result of spontaneous mutations, engineered mutations introduced by transgenesis or gene targeting, radiation, or chemical-induced mutations. The mapping and identification of genetic modifiers is easier in laboratory animals such as the mouse, as a number of variables can be controlled by maintaining environmental conditions and controlled breeding, factors that otherwise could interfere with the phenotypic manifestation. The genetic bases for modification in most cases are unknown. But, in a few cases, genetic modifiers have been mapped, phenotypically evaluated, and the causal variants identified (table 1).

dfw
The deafwaddler (dfw) recessive mutation arose spontaneously in a C3H/HeJ mouse colony and was mapped to chromosome 6. Homozygous dfw mice exhibit hesitant and wobbly gait along with head bobbing and hearing loss [26, 27]. Subsequently, a second dfw allele (dfw^{2J}) was identified on a BALB/cBy genetic background [28]. Eventually, mutations in the Atp2b2 gene, encoding plasma membrane Ca^{2+} ATPase 2 (PMCA2), were identified as responsible for the dfw phenotype [29]. PMCA2 is a pump involved in clearing the Ca^{2+} from the hair cell stereocilia into the endolymph [29].

Table 1. Summary of genetic modifiers of inherited hearing loss identified in mice

Disease phenotype	Disease allele		Genetic modifier		Phenotypic modification	Reference
	locus	gene	locus	gene		
Wobbly gait, head bobbing, and hearing loss	dfw	Atp2b2	mdfw	potentially Cdh23	CAST/Ei genetic background prevents hearing loss	[26–28]
Heterozygous dfw²ᴶ mice on BALB/cBy exhibit hearing loss	dfw²ᴶ	Atp2b2	mdfw	potentially Cdh23	CAST/Ei genetic background prevents hearing loss	[28, 30]
Obesity, insulin resistance, retina and cochlear degeneration	tub	Tub	moth1	Mtap1a	AKR/J, CAST/Ei and 129P2/Ola mice genetic background prevents hearing loss	[31–33]
Hypothyroidism and hearing loss	DW/J-Pou1f1ᵈʷ/ᵈʷ	Pou1f1	Mdwh	unknown	CAST/EiJ genetic background reduces hearing loss penetrance	[34]
Human branchiootorenal (BOR) syndrome, including hearing loss	Eya1ᵇᵒʳ/ᵇᵒʳ	Eya1	Mead1, Mead2	unknown	suppression of the hearing loss phenotype	[35]

Intriguingly, heterozygous dfw^{2J} mice on BALB/cBy background also exhibited progressive hearing loss starting at 4 weeks and were completely deaf by 12 weeks of age [28]. The hearing loss in heterozygous dfw^{2J} mice appeared to be dependent on the genetic background. Linkage analysis mapped the locus of a modifier of deafwaddler (mdfw) to chromosome 10 [28]. The Cdh23 gene, responsible for deafness and vestibular dysfunction in waltzer mice, also resides in close proximity to the mdfw locus, suggesting the possibility that the mdfw and waltzer phenotypes are caused by allelic variants [30]. However, experimental evidence is still needed to directly verify that alleles of Cdh23 are responsible for mdfw-based phenotypic variations.

Tubby

Homozygous mutations in the neuronal tub gene are responsible for maturity onset obesity, along with retinal and cochlear degeneration in mice [31]. However, the hearing loss associated with tub/tub on C57Bl/6 strain background mice is completely rescued in F2 progeny when outcrossed so that the genetic background is derived from AKR/J, CAST/Ei or 129P2/Ola mouse strains. Quantitative trait locus (QTL) analysis identified a modifier locus 'modifier of tubby hearing 1 (moth1)' on chromosome 2 [32]. A mutation in the neuron-specific microtubule-associated protein 1a gene (Mtap1a) was identified at the moth1 locus in the susceptible strain C57BL/6J. The mutation affects the binding efficiency of MTAP1A to postsynaptic density molecule 95 (PSD95), a protein that is a major component of the synaptic junction [33]. The fact that TUB is involved in vesicular trafficking and G-protein coupled receptor [33], which are also present in synaptic junctions of neuronal cells, suggests that Mtap1a may exert its modifying effect at the synaptic junctions between hair cells and cochlear neurons [33].

DW/J-Pou1f1ᵈʷ/ᵈʷ

Thyroid hormones are critical for the proper development and physiology of the cochlea. DW/J-Pou1f1ᵈʷ/ᵈʷ mutant mice exhibit a thyroid

Table 2. Summary of genetic modifiers of inherited hearing loss identified in humans

Disease phenotype	Disease allele		Genetic modifier		Phenotypic modification of hearing	Reference
	locus	gene	locus	gene		
Nonsyndromic sensorineural hearing loss	DFNB26	unknown	DFNM1	unknown	completely rescues hearing loss	[36]
	mitochondrial A1555G	12S rRNA	DFNM2	unknown	exacerbates severity of hearing loss	[38, 39]
			–	MTO1/GTPBP3	exacerbates severity of hearing loss	[40]
			–	TRMU	exacerbates severity of hearing loss	[41]
Autosomal recessive nonsyndromic hearing loss	DFNB1	GJB2	–	unknown	modulates hearing loss, ranging from mild to profound	[45–47]
	DFNB12	CDH23	–	ATP2B2	increased severity of hearing loss	[48]

hormone deficiency along with profound hearing loss. However, when intercrossed with the CAST/EiJ inbred mouse strain, 24% of the offspring had normal hearing [34]. Further analysis of these hearing mice revealed a modifier of dw hearing (*Mdwh*) locus on chromosome 2, which rescued the hearing loss, albeit not the hypothyroidism [34]. Additional studies are required to identify the causative mutant allele at the *Mdwh* locus.

Eya1
Another example of a genetic modifier comes from studies of the *Eya1^bor^* mutant mouse. This is a recessive mouse model for human branchiootorenal (BOR) syndrome, which exhibits hearing loss and other clinical phenotypes such as branchial fistulas or cysts, and renal abnormalities. The severity of the hearing phenotype depends on the genetic background of the mouse [35]. An intercross between C3HeB/FeJ-*Eya1^bor/+^* and C57BL/6J showed variable auditory brainstem responses and reduced cochlear turns. QTL analysis in F$_2$ *Eya1^bor/bor^* mutants identified 2 modifier loci, *Mead1* and *Mead2* (modifier of Eya1-associ-

ated deafness 1 and 2), mapping to chromosomes 4 and 12, respectively, that were able to partially suppress the original hearing loss phenotype. However, the identity of the modifier genes and their mechanisms of action are unknown [35].

Modifiers of Hearing Loss in Humans

Table 2 lists the reported genetic modifiers associated with hearing loss in humans that are briefly discussed here. The first example is from work by the authors of this review.

DFNM1
The *DFNB26* locus was genetically mapped in a large consanguineous Pakistani family to chromosome 4q31. The family was segregating prelingual, nonsyndromic sensorineural hearing loss [36]. Eight affected individuals in the family had severe to profound hearing loss. Intriguingly, besides the 8 deaf individuals, 7 additional family members were homozygous for the *DFNB26*-linked haplotype, but had normal hearing (fig. 1).

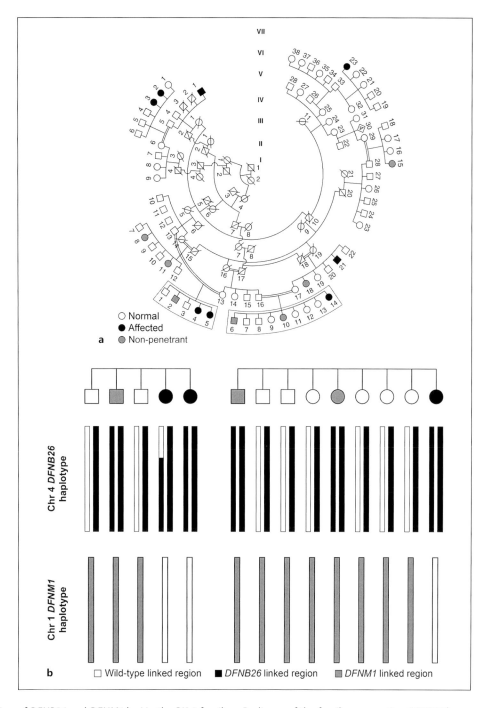

Fig. 1. Segregation of *DFNB26* and *DFNM1* loci in the PK-2 family. **a** Pedigree of the family segregating *DFNB26* hearing loss and the *DFNM1* modifier gene. Black symbols are deaf individuals homozygous for the *DFNB26*-linked haplotype. Gray symbols are normal hearing, non-penetrant individuals homozygous for *DFNB26* haplotype and also carrying the modifier allele at chromosome 1. **b** Schematic representation of digenic inheritance of *DFNB26* (black) and *DFNM1* (gray) linked haplotypes on chromosomes 4 and 1, respectively, for the framed sibships in panel **a**.

These non-penetrant individuals were used in a linkage study to map the modifier. This work revealed a dominant modifier locus, *DFNM1*, on chromosome 1q24. The 7 non-penetrant individuals carried the *DFNM1* haplotype while the 8 deaf individuals did not carry the *DFNM1* haplotype (fig. 1). The variant responsible for the *DFNM1* suppressor of *DFNB26* has not yet been reported. We speculated that *DFNM1* and dominantly inherited nonsyndromic hearing loss *DFNA7* [37], also mapped to chromosome 1, are caused by allelic variants. *DFNM1* was the first hearing loss suppressor described in humans [36]. The obvious question arises as to whether or not the mechanism of action of the variant underlying the *DFNM1* modifier may be a general modifier of other types of human inherited hearing loss and not just suppression of *DFNB26* deafness.

DFNM2

DFNM2 was the second reported modifier of human inherited hearing loss. The A1555G mutation in the mitochondrial 12S rRNA gene was the first mitochondrial mutation identified to cause nonsyndromic hearing loss in humans, with a maternal mode of transmission [38]. Phenotypic variation in the hearing loss associated with this mutation ranges from profound congenital deafness to progressive moderate hearing loss starting in adult life to normal hearing. Moreover, the A1555G mutation also predisposes individuals to aminoglycoside-induced hearing loss [38]. Biochemical and genetic analyses are highly suggestive that there are nuclear genetic factors as the cause of the phenotypic differences among the families segregating the mitochondrial A1555G variant [39].

The nuclear modifier gene for the *DFNM2* locus on chromosome 8 has not yet been identified. However, some nuclear genes that encode mitochondrial proteins, such as TFB1M, which is involved in the methylation of mitochondrial 12S rRNA, have been proposed to modify the hearing loss associated with the mitochondrial A1555G mutation. Additionally, variants of *MTO1* and *GTPBP3* have been implicated in the mitochondrial transfer RNA (tRNA) modification machinery [40]. Recently, *TRMU*, another nuclear modifier gene, was shown to exacerbate the hearing loss associated with the mitochondrial A1555G mutation. Functional studies have demonstrated that substitution p.Ala10Ser of TRMU results in defective mitochondrial tRNA metabolism, reducing the steady-state levels of mitochondrial tRNA. The presence of p.Ala10Ser further worsens the hearing loss phenotype associated with the mitochondrial A1555G mutation [41].

GJB2

GJB2 encodes a gap junction protein, connexin 26, at the *DFNB1* locus. Depending on ethnicity, mutations of *GJB2* account for as much as 50% of the autosomal recessive nonsyndromic hearing loss cases [42]. To date, 236 mutant alleles have been identified for *GJB2*, segregating in different world populations. Among them, the c.35delG allele accounts for 70% of *GJB2* mutations in the European population [43], while c.167delT is the major cause of nonsyndromic hearing loss among Ashkenazi Jews [44]. Both c.35delG and c.167delT mutant alleles have been shown to exhibit significant intra- and interfamilial variation in the severity of the phenotypic manifestation, ranging from mild to profound hearing loss [45, 46]. Although attempts have been made to map the genetic modifier, no major locus has been identified, suggesting that the modifier may arise from the combination of multiple etiologies, perhaps each alone imparting only a small impact on the hearing loss phenotype [47].

CDH23

Genes can reciprocally modulate each other's phenotype. For example, in a family segregating autosomal recessive sensorineural hearing loss, genetic analysis revealed homozygous changes in *CDH23* to be the likely cause in all 5 affected siblings. However, 2 affected members of the family had only high-frequency loss, whereas the other 3 had severe-to-profound loss across all frequencies. Further genetic analyses identified a heterozygous hypofunctional variant in the PMCA2 (ATP2B2) gene, which in 3 severely affected siblings was associated with increased severity of hearing loss [48]. Interestingly, the *Cdh23* allele is believed to modify the hearing loss phenotype in *Pmca2* mutant mice [30], which suggests that the allelic state of these 2 genes can interact to modify the phenotypic outcome of the other.

Phenotypic Variability Potentially due to Modifier Genes

In most instances, a single major gene is the sole cause of hearing loss. However, severity or onset of hearing loss sometimes cannot be attributed to the variant of a single gene alone, but rather are modified by other variants that have not been genetically identified, however, nevertheless detected phenotypically.

TRIC

The *DFNB49* locus was genetically mapped in 2 Pakistani families segregating nonsyndromic hearing loss. The *DFNB49* locus encompasses an 11-cM interval on chromosome 5q12.3q14.1 [49]. This linkage interval was refined to 2.4 Mb after ascertaining additional *DFNB49*-linked families. Within the refined linkage interval, *TRIC* (also referred to as *MARVELD2*) was identified to harbor a number of allelic variants, which included several splice site alleles and a nonsense mutation in exons 4 and 5, all resulting in premature truncation of the tricellulin protein [50]. Pure tone air conduction of *DFNB49*-affected individuals from 7 different families revealed marked intra- and interfamilial variability, which did not correlate with age of onset, sex or allelic variants [50]. A subsequent study identified more families segregating *TRIC* mutant alleles which exhibited variability in the severity of the hearing loss similar to that previously reported [51]. This observed phenotypic variability could plausibly stem from genetic modifiers, environmental factors or both.

CLDN14

Tricellulin and claudin 14 are tight junction-associated transmembrane proteins. Mutations of *CLDN14* encoding claudin 14 are responsible for causing autosomal recessive nonsyndromic hearing loss mapped to the *DFNB29* locus. In an effort to identify the frequency and identity of *CLDN14* mutations, hearing loss in a large cohort of Pakistani families segregating autosomal recessive nonsyndromic hearing loss was examined. Five different pathogenic alleles of *CLDN14* were identified segregating in 15 unrelated families [52]. Furthermore, analysis of pure tone air and bone conduction audiometry of the affected individuals in these families revealed inter- and intrafamilial variability in the severity of hearing loss that did not correlate with age or the associated pathogenic variant. Genetic modifiers are potentially involved. Claudin 14 is a member of a family of tight junction proteins, and in the inner ear tight junctions are complex and composed of a great variety of proteins. Perhaps upregulation of one of the other tight junction proteins would partially suppress the deleterious deafness-causing effect of a mutation in *CLDN14*. Variation in the expression levels of several tight junction proteins in the inner ear might alter the degree of hearing loss due to a damaging mutation in one of these genes.

Modifier Alleles

MYO7A

Mutations of *MYO7A* can result in either recessive (DFNB2) or dominant (DFNA11) forms of inherited nonsyndromic hearing loss, while other mutations of *MYO7A* cause Usher syndrome type 1, characterized by hearing loss which is often profound at birth, a progressive loss of vision due to retinitis pigmentosa and vestibular areflexia [53]. A p.Gly2164Cys mutation of *MYO7A* results in nonsyndromic hearing loss initially affecting the low and mid frequencies. A high degree of phenotypic variability was observed in a family segregating this mutant allele, which suggests a genetic modifier that either enhances or suppresses the effect of the primary *MYO7A* p.Gly2164Cys mutation [54]. A single nucleotide polymorphism (SNP) T/C at position –4128 (rs10899353) was identified in the wild-type *MYO7A* promoter, which co-segregates with the degree of hearing loss severity observed in the family. Experimental evidence suggests that the SNP reduces the binding of the *YY1* transcription factor to the *MYO7A* promoter. This results in a reduced expression of *MYO7A*, which was suggested to enhance hearing loss [55].

Mcoln3

The varitint-waddler (*Va*) mice exhibit early-onset hearing loss, vestibular dysfunction, pigmentation defects, and perinatal lethality. By contrast, a second allele *Va^J^* arose in the *Va* mouse line, exhibiting a less severe phenotype. Whereas, *Va^J^*/*Va^J^* and +/*Va^J^* mutants both show impaired cochlear function with no detectable compound action potential and with small or absent endocochlear potentials. Mice with the +/*Va^J^* allele exhibit a milder phenotype, with normal vestibular function, some residual hearing, and limited variation of coat color [56, 57]. However, *Va^J^*/*Va^J^* and +/*Va* mice exhibit similar phenotypes with intermediate penetrance and having defects in the sensory epithelium and hypopigmentation in melanocytes located in the stria vascularis [57].

Mcoln3 was identified as the causative gene in varitint-waddler mice through a positional cloning strategy. *Mcoln3* encodes a transmembrane-domain protein. The *Va* mouse has a p.Ala419Pro substitution in the 5th transmembrane domain, and in the *Va^J^* mice, p.Ile362Thr occurred in *cis*

partially rescuing the *Va* allele phenotype [58]. This is an example of a modifier allele working in *cis* with the mutant allele of the same gene.

Identification of New Genetic Modifiers

For many Mendelian disorders, a particular variant of a gene can predictably cause a specific disease phenotype, and the environment seems to play no role in the severity. But for many inherited disorders, the environment, epigenetic marks and modifier variants in the genome contribute to the phenotypic outcome. The first step toward an understanding of pathophysiology of modifiers is the identification of the DNA sequence(s) responsible for phenotypic modulation. However, before embarking on a mapping project of genetic modifiers, it is imperative to consider other possibilities such as nongenetic or stochastic factors that could potentially be responsible for phenotypic variability.

Mapping and identification of genetic modifiers in humans has proven to be extremely difficult due to multiple factors, including genetic heterogeneity and sample size. However, genetic analyses of inbred populations and extended human pedigrees can be useful for mapping modifiers of hearing loss. Mapping the *DFNM1* locus to an interval on chromosome 1q23 in a large consanguineous family segregating DFNB26-linked hearing loss [36], and mapping *DFNM2* to chromosome 8p23 in Arab-Israeli, Spanish and Italian families segregating the mitochondrial A1555G pathogenic allele-associated hearing loss [59] are some examples.

An alternate approach to identify genetic modifiers is through genome-wide association studies. Recently, such a study has been undertaken to assess the role of genetic modifier(s) in phenotype variability for hearing loss observed in individuals homozygous for the c.35delG allele of *GJB2* [47]. However, analyses of 1,277 individuals from 14 countries did not reveal a major genetic modifier locus associated with the observed phenotypic variability [47]. Therefore, the cumulative effect of multiple loci (locus heterogeneity) was suggested as the cause of hearing loss variability associated with the c.35delG allele of *GJB2* [47].

Current advancements in massive parallel sequencing technologies (MPS) have resulted in rapid identification of genetic mutations for many Mendelian disorders, including hearing loss [60, 61]. Although MPS has helped make headway in the identification of causal variants in simple to slightly complex Mendelian disorders, so far a modifier of hearing loss has not been identified using MPS.

In a yet another alternate approach, Jordan et al. [62] used a comparative genomics approach to parse out the compensatory alleles that are modifying disease causing alleles. Evolutionarily, the sequences that are conserved during evolution are more likely to resist change. However, an allele may appear damaging in humans, but be neutral in the orthologous sequence of another species as a result of compensation exerted by variants elsewhere in their genetic background. Jordan et al. [62] functionally tested this model on 2 known human disease genes causing ciliopathies and found compensatory mutations that modify the pathogenic alleles in vivo. Moreover, they were able to rescue the phenotype by protective *cis*-modification in the de novo disease allele

identified in the *BTG2* gene in the zebrafish model system [62]. Recently, in *C. elegans* another example of a genetic background effect on the penetrance of a phenotype has been reported [63]. Vu et al. [63] performed massive loss-of-function analyses for 1,353 genes in 2 different isolates of *C. elegans* and found that ~20% of the genes varied significantly in the penetrance between isolates, owing to the differences in their genetic architecture. These findings emphasize the significance of the combinatorial effect of variants, in addition to the major disease-causing allele.

Conclusion

The study of genetic modifiers, especially suppressors, will provide insights into the mechanisms by which organisms can accommodate the adverse effects of genetic mutations. Modifier effects could be a result of an interaction between only 2 proteins or a complex of several macromolecules that have a combined effect, in which case identifying such genetic modifiers will be challenging. Studying genetic modifiers will help us to understand the complex molecular and functional landscape involved in the pathophysiology of disease and its phenotypic modulation. Moreover, characterization of genetic modifiers should help with the development of new therapeutic targets to prevent hearing loss.

References

1 World Health Organization: Deafness and hearing loss. Fact sheet 300, updated February 2014. http://www.who.int/mediacentre/factsheets/fs300/en/ (accessed January 16, 2015).
2 Morton CC, Nance WE: Newborn hearing screening – a silent revolution. New Engl J Med 2006;354:2151–2164.
3 Lim DJ: Effects of noise and ototoxic drugs at the cellular level in the cochlea: a review. Am J Otolaryngol 1986;7:73–99.
4 Fowler KB, McCollister FP, Dahle AJ, Boppana S, Britt WJ, Pass RF: Progressive and fluctuating sensorineural hearing loss in children with asymptomatic congenital cytomegalovirus infection. J Pediatr 1997;130:624–630.
5 McCabe BF: Autoimmune sensorineural hearing loss. Ann Otol Rhinol Laryngol 1979;88:585–589.
6 Gorlin RJ, Toriello HV, Cohen MM: Hereditary Hearing Loss and Its Syndromes. New York, Oxford University Press, 1995.
7 Angeli S, Lin X, Liu XZ: Genetics of hearing and deafness. Anat Rec 2012; 295:1812–1829.
8 Lenz DR, Avraham KB: Hereditary hearing loss: from human mutation to mechanism. Hear Res 2011;281:3–10.

9 Friedman TB, Griffith AJ: Human non-syndromic sensorineural deafness. Ann Rev Genomics Hum Genet 2003;4:341–402.

10 Ruben R: Bacterial meningitic deafness: historical development of epidemiology and cellular pathology. Acta Otolaryngol 2008;128:388–392.

11 Federspil P: Drug-induced sudden hearing loss and vestibular disturbances. Adv Otorhinolaryngol 1981;27:144–158.

12 Wheeler DE: Noise-induced hearing loss. Arch Otolaryngol 1950;51:344–355.

13 Rosen S, Olin P, Rosen HV: Diery prevention of hearing loss. Acta Otolaryngol 1970;70:242–247.

14 Castle WE: The inconstancy of unit-characters. Am Nat 1912;46:352–362.

15 Castle WE: Further studies of piebald rats and selection, with observations on gametic coupling. Carnegie Inst Wash Publ 1916;241:163–192.

16 Dipple KM, McCabe ER: Phenotypes of patients with 'simple' Mendelian disorders are complex traits: thresholds, modifiers, and systems dynamics. Am J Hum Genet 2000;66:1729–1735.

17 Nadeau JH: Modifier genes in mice and humans. Nat Rev Genet 2001;2:165–174.

18 Ming JE, Muenke M: Multiple hits during early embryonic development: digenic diseases and holoprosencephaly. Am J Hum Genet 2002;71:1017–1032.

19 Weatherall DJ: Phenotype-genotype relationships in monogenic disease: lessons from the thalassaemias. Nat Rev Genet 2001;2:245–255.

20 Nadeau JH, Topol EJ: The genetics of health. Nat Genet 2006;38:1095–1098.

21 Haider NB, Ikeda A, Naggert JK, Nishina PM: Genetic modifiers of vision and hearing. Hum Mol Genet 2002;11:1195–1206.

22 Utz VM, Beight CD, Marino MJ, Hagstrom SA, Traboulsi EI: Autosomal dominant retinitis pigmentosa secondary to pre-mRNA splicing-factor gene *PRPF31* (RP11): review of disease mechanism and report of a family with a novel 3-base pair insertion. Ophthalmic Genet 2013;34:183–188.

23 Vithana EN, Abu-Safieh L, Pelosini L, Winchester E, Hornan D, et al: Expression of *PRPF31* mRNA in patients with autosomal dominant retinitis pigmentosa: a molecular clue for incomplete penetrance? Invest Ophthalmol Vis Sci 2003;44:4204–4209.

24 Venturini G, Rose AM, Shah AZ, Bhattacharya SS, Rivolta C: *CNOT3* is a modifier of *PRPF31* mutations in retinitis pigmentosa with incomplete penetrance. PLoS Genet 2012;8:e1003040.

25 Johnson KR, Zheng QY, Noben-Trauth K: Strain background effects and genetic modifiers of hearing in mice. Brain Res 2006;1091:79–88.

26 Lane PW: New mutants and linkages: deafwaddler *(dfw)*. Mouse News Lett 1987;77:129.

27 Street VA, Robinson LC, Erford SK, Tempel BL: Molecular genetic analysis of distal mouse chromosome 6 defines gene order and positions of the deafwaddler and opisthotonos mutations. Genomics 1995;29:123–130.

28 Noben-Trauth K, Zheng QY, Johnson KR, Nishina PM: *mdfw*: a deafness susceptibility locus that interacts with deaf waddler *(dfw)*. Genomics 1997;44:266–272.

29 Street VA, McKee-Johnson JW, Fonseca RC, Tempel BL, Noben-Trauth K: Mutations in a plasma membrane Ca^{2+}-ATPase gene cause deafness in deafwaddler mice. Nat Genet 1998;19:390–394.

30 Di Palma F, Holme RH, Bryda EC, Belyantseva IA, Pellegrino R, et al: Mutations in *Cdh23*, encoding a new type of cadherin, cause stereocilia disorganization in waltzer, the mouse model for Usher syndrome type 1D. Nat Genet 2001;27:103–107.

31 Ohlemiller KK, Hughes RM, Lett JM, Ogilvie JM, Speck JD, et al: Progression of cochlear and retinal degeneration in the tubby (rd5) mouse. Audiol Neurotol 1997;2:175–185.

32 Ikeda A, Zheng QY, Rosenstiel P, Maddatu T, Zuberi AR, et al: Genetic modification of hearing in tubby mice: evidence for the existence of a major gene *(moth1)* which protects tubby mice from hearing loss. Hum Mol Genet 1999;8:1761–1767.

33 Ikeda A, Nishina PM, Naggert JK: The tubby-like proteins, a family with roles in neuronal development and function. J Cell Sci 2002;115:9–14.

34 Fang Q, Longo-Guess C, Gagnon LH, Mortensen AH, Dolan DF, et al: A modifier gene alleviates hypothyroidism-induced hearing impairment in *Pou1f1^dw* dwarf mice. Genetics 2011;189:665–673.

35 Niu H, Makmura L, Shen T, Sheth SS, Blair K, Friedman RA: Identification of two major loci that suppress hearing loss and cochlear dysmorphogenesis in *Eya1^bor/bor* mice. Genomics 2006;88:302–308.

36 Riazuddin S, Castelein CM, Ahmed ZM, Lalwani AK, Mastroianni MA, et al: Dominant modifier *DFNM1* suppresses recessive deafness *DFNB26*. Nat Genet 2000;26:431–434.

37 Fagerheim T, Nilssen O, Raeymaekers P, Brox V, Moum T, et al: Identification of a new locus for autosomal dominant non-syndromic hearing impairment *(DFNA7)* in a large Norwegian family. Hum Mol Genet 1996;5:1187–1191.

38 Prezant TR, Agapian JV, Bohlman MC, Bu X, Oztas S, et al: Mitochondrial ribosomal RNA mutation associated with both antibiotic-induced and non-syndromic deafness. Nat Genet 1993;4:289–294.

39 Guan MX, Fischel-Ghodsian N, Attardi G: Biochemical evidence for nuclear gene involvement in phenotype of non-syndromic deafness associated with mitochondrial 12S rRNA mutation. Hum Mol Genet 1996;5:963–971.

40 Bykhovskaya Y, Mengesha E, Wang D, Yang H, Estivill X, et al: Phenotype of non-syndromic deafness associated with the mitochondrial A1555G mutation is modulated by mitochondrial RNA modifying enzymes *MTO1* and *GTPBP3*. Mol Genet Metab 2004;83:199–206.

41 Guan MX, Yan Q, Li X, Bykhovskaya Y, Gallo-Teran J, et al: Mutation in *TRMU* related to transfer RNA modification modulates the phenotypic expression of the deafness-associated mitochondrial 12S ribosomal RNA mutations. Am J Hum Genet 2006;79:291–302.

42 Kenneson A, Van Naarden Braun K, Boyle C: GJB2 (connexin 26) variants and nonsyndromic sensorineural hearing loss: a HuGE review. Genet Med 2002;4:258–274.

43 Gasparini P, Rabionet R, Barbujani G, Melchionda S, Petersen M, et al: High carrier frequency of the 35delG deafness mutation in European populations. Genetic Analysis Consortium of *GJB2* 35delG. Eur J Hum Genet 2000;8:19–23.

44 Sobe T, Vreugde S, Shahin H, Berlin M, Davis N, et al: The prevalence and expression of inherited connexin 26 mutations associated with nonsyndromic hearing loss in the Israeli population. Hum Genet 2000;106:50–57.

45 Cohn ES, Kelley PM, Fowler TW, Gorga MP, Lefkowitz DM, et al: Clinical studies of families with hearing loss attributable to mutations in the connexin 26 gene (GJB2/DFNB1). Pediatrics 1999;103: 546–550.

46 Azaiez H, Chamberlin GP, Fischer SM, Welp CL, Prasad SD, et al: *GJB2*: the spectrum of deafness-causing allele variants and their phenotype. Hum Mutat 2004;24:305–311.

47 Hilgert N, Huentelman MJ, Thorburn AQ, Fransen E, Dieltjens N, et al: Phenotypic variability of patients homozygous for the *GJB2* mutation 35delG cannot be explained by the influence of one major modifier gene. Eur J Hum Genet 2009; 17:517–524.

48 Schultz JM, Yang Y, Caride AJ, Filoteo AG, Penheiter AR, et al: Modification of human hearing loss by plasma-membrane calcium pump PMCA2. New Engl J Med 2005;352:1557–1764.

49 Ramzan K, Shaikh RS, Ahmad J, Khan SN, Riazuddin S, et al: A new locus for nonsyndromic deafness *DFNB49* maps to chromosome 5q12.3-q14.1. Hum Genet 2005;116:17–22.

50 Riazuddin S, Ahmed ZM, Fanning AS, Lagziel A, Kitajiri S, et al: Tricellulin is a tight-junction protein necessary for hearing. Am J Hum Genet 2006;79: 1040–1051.

51 Nayak G, Varga L, Trincot C, Shahzad M, Friedman PL, et al: Molecular genetics of *MARVELD2* and clinical phenotype in Pakistani and Slovak families segregating DFNB49 hearing loss. Hum Genet 2015;134:423–437.

52 Bashir ZE, Latief N, Belyantseva IA, Iqbal F, Riazuddin SA, et al: Phenotypic variability of *CLDN14* mutations causing DFNB29 hearing loss in the Pakistani population. J Hum Genet 2013;58:102–108.

53 Weil D, Kussel P, Blanchard S, Levy G, Levi-Acobas F, et al: The autosomal recessive isolated deafness, DFNB2, and the Usher 1B syndrome are allelic defects of the myosin-VIIA gene. Nat Genet 1997;16:191–193.

54 Street VA, Kallman JC, Kiemele KL: Modifier controls severity of a novel dominant low-frequency MyosinVIIA *(MYO7A)* auditory mutation. J Med Genet 2004;41:e62.

55 Street VA, Li J, Robbins CA, Kallman JC: A DNA variant within the *MYO7A* promoter regulates YY1 transcription factor binding and gene expression serving as a potential dominant *DFNA11* auditory genetic modifier. J Biol Chem 2011;286: 15278–15286.

56 Lane PW: Two new mutations in linkage group XVI of the house mouse. Flaky tail and varitint-waddler-J. J Hered 1972;63:135–140.

57 Cable J, Steel KP: Combined cochleosaccular and neuroepithelial abnormalities in the Varitint-waddler-J *(Va^J)* mouse. Hear Res 1998;123:125–136.

58 Di Palma F, Belyantseva IA, Kim HJ, Vogt TF, Kachar B, Noben-Trauth K: Mutations in *Mcoln3* associated with deafness and pigmentation defects in varitint-waddler *(Va)* mice. Proc Natl Acad Sci U S A 2002;99:14994–14999.

59 Bykhovskaya Y, Estivill X, Taylor K, Hang T, Hamon M, et al: Candidate locus for a nuclear modifier gene for maternally inherited deafness. Am J Hum Genet 2000;66:1905–1910.

60 Rehman AU, Morell RJ, Belyantseva IA, Khan SY, Boger ET, et al: Targeted capture and next-generation sequencing identifies *C9orf75*, encoding taperin, as the mutated gene in nonsyndromic deafness DFNB79. Am J Hum Genet 2010;86:378–388.

61 Walsh T, Shahin H, Elkan-Miller T, Lee MK, Thornton AM, et al: Whole exome sequencing and homozygosity mapping identify mutation in the cell polarity protein GPSM2 as the cause of nonsyndromic hearing loss DFNB82. Am J Hum Genet 2010;87:90–94.

62 Jordan DM, Frangakis SG, Golzio C, Cassa CA, Kurtzberg J, et al: Identification of *cis*-suppression of human disease mutations by comparative genomics. Nature 2015;524:225–229.

63 Vu V, Verster AJ, Schertzberg M, Chuluunbaatar T, Spensley M, et al: Natural variation in gene expression modulates the severity of mutant phenotypes. Cell 2015;162:391–402.

Saima Riazuddin, MBA, MPH, PhD
Department of Otorhinolaryngology – Head and Neck Surgery
School of Medicine, University of Maryland
BioPark1, 800 West Baltimore St., 400-L
Baltimore, MD 21201 (USA)
E-Mail sriazuddin@smail.umaryland.edu

Vona B, Haaf T (eds): Genetics of Deafness. Monogr Hum Genet. Basel, Karger, 2016, vol 20, pp 84–96
(DOI: 10.1159/000444565)

Genetics of Age-Related Hearing Loss

Piers Dawes · Antony Payton

School of Psychological Sciences, The University of Manchester, Manchester, UK

Abstract

Age-related hearing loss (ARHL) is a complex multifactorial disease. It is highly prevalent in older adults and has significant adverse impact on communication, mental health and quality of life. Severity and onset of ARHL varies substantially between individuals, and heritability estimates of ARHL range up to 75%. Understanding the genetics of ARHL may allow targeted treatment or prevention. We review the current research in humans on genetic susceptibility to ARHL related to (1) cell adhesion, cell shape and epithelial development, (2) neurotransmission, (3) oxidative stress, (4) immune response/apoptosis, and (5) other functions.   © 2016 S. Karger AG, Basel

Age-related hearing loss (ARHL) or 'presbycusis' is very common [1]. The clinical level of hearing loss (a hearing threshold in the better ear ≥25 dB HL over 0.5 to 4 kHz) in the age range between 71 and 80 years is estimated at 60% [2]. With aging populations, the number of people with ARHL in developed countries is increasing. Hearing loss is associated with communication difficulties, social isolation, cognitive decline, and reduced physical and emotional well-being [3]. The high prevalence, increasing proportion of the population affected and impact of ARHL on quality of life result in substantial burden to society. One report concluded that hearing loss costs Europe 213 billion Euros per year [4]. Similar high costs have been estimated for the US [5]. Hearing loss is set to be in the top 10 disease burdens in high- and middle-income countries by 2030 [6]. The primary treatment for ARHL is provision of hearing aids, although uptake of hearing aids is limited due to negative stigma, uncomfortable fit, limited benefit, and cost [7].

Understanding the genetics of ARHL is therefore of interest, because insight into the genetics of ARHL may indicate the most significant biological pathways and thus allow targeted treatment and/or prevention. There is wide variability between individuals in the onset and severity of ARHL [8], and ARHL appears to have a strong genetic contribution. Estimates of heritability of ARHL range between 25 and 75%, depending on the ARHL phenotype measure and the study population [9–12]. We will review the biology of ARHL and the implications for ARHL genetics, summarise current genetic findings of ARHL in humans, and conclude with suggestions for future directions.

The Biology of ARHL

ARHL is a complex disorder, in terms of both pathology and aetiology. A variety of pathological changes are associated with ARHL. Schuknecht compared histological analyses of human inner ears with pre-mortem hearing tests [13, 14] and described 4 primary types of pathology; (1) sensory; loss of outer hair cells characterised by high-frequency audiometric losses; (2) neural; degeneration of the auditory nerve, characterised by poor speech recognition; (3) strial; degeneration of the stria vascularis leading to flat audiometric losses across frequencies; and (4) cochlear conductive; a hypothetical category associated with increased stiffness of the basilar membrane resulting in evenly sloping audiometric losses. Analyses of large numbers of audiograms found that most audiograms lie in between extremes of either flat or sloping high frequency loss, suggesting that most cases of ARHL may involve a mixture of changes described by Schuknecht [15]. Uncertainties remain whether particular pathological types such as those described by Schuknecht can be mapped onto a characteristic audiometric profile [16], although Schuknecht's work remains influential in understanding pathologies underlying ARHL. Different types of hearing pathology may have different levels of heritability. Based on analysis of audiometric shapes, Gates et al. [10] reported that heritability was greater for strial than sensory type hearing loss. Huyghe et al. [17] also reported greater heritability for a flat audiometric shape characteristic of overall 'severity'

(which might be consistent with strial hearing loss), with lower heritability for a steeply sloping high frequency hearing loss (characteristic of sensory loss).

If different types of ARHL pathology do have different genetic contributions, the method of measuring the phenotype of ARHL may be critical for human ARHL genetic research. To date, most studies have used self-report or average audiometric hearing threshold over selected frequencies. Self-reported hearing problems is a quick and inexpensive measure, but self-report may underestimate actual cases of hearing loss, provides no indication of severity or underlying pathology, and results in a significant loss of statistical power for genetic analyses. A recent approach to describing phenotypes of ARHL involved applying principal component (PC) analysis (PCA) to audiograms to provide PC values for each participant [17]. PCA resulted in PC scores for 3 components; 'severity', 'slope' and 'concavity'. The audiometric shapes derived by PCA may relate to different underlying pathologies, although the authors of this method did not explicitly describe which PCs might relate to particular types of hearing loss. One limitation of audiogram-based phenotype measures is that audiometry may not be sensitive to neural type hearing loss [1]. Measures of speech recognition in noise are sensitive to neural hearing loss, and speech recognition tests have been used in recent ARHL genetics studies [18–21]. In a twin study using both audiometric and speech recognition test data, speech recognition data correlated strongly with audiometric data [18]. But higher estimates of heritability were obtained for audiometric versus speech recognition-based phenotypes, suggesting that although audiometric and speech recognition-based tests may overlap, they could provide complementary information about the genetic contribution to different underlying pathologies of ARHL.

In terms of aetiology, ARHL reflects age-related changes overlaid with the effects of cumulative noise damage and other environmental insults such as ototoxic drugs, smoking and diet [1]. Age-related processes that may impact hearing include oxidative stress and damage to mitochondrial DNA which may be exacerbated by age-related reductions in the blood supply to the cochlea [22, 23] and ionic dysregulation resulting in loss of endocochlear potential [24]. Noise-induced hearing loss (NIHL) occurs as a result of damage to hair cells of the inner ear and is characterised by an audiometric 'notch' at 3–4 kHz, with some recovery of thresholds at 8 kHz [25]. Short-duration high intensity sound such as gunshots can cause immediate structural damage to the cochlea, while more prolonged exposure to lower sound levels causes metabolic disruption, whose effects may continue for days or weeks after the original exposure. Genetic research primarily with mouse models has identified various genetic susceptibility factors for NIHL [26]. Confounding of ARHL with NIHL makes it a challenging task to separate genetic susceptibility factors associated with age rather than with susceptibility to noise. It is not straightforward to distinguish NIHL from ARHL based on the audiogram. The audiometric 'notch' that is characteristic of NIHL is easier to identify in younger adults with otherwise good hearing, but with aging the notch tends to broaden and become subsumed within audiometric losses across frequencies. It might be possible to observe 'pure' ARHL in animal models which can be protected from noise exposure, or in human societies with low levels of industrial or recreational noise exposure. However, most people growing up in a society with high levels of noise are likely to have at least some NIHL.

ARHL is also associated with a range of lifestyle and environmental factors such as smoking [27, 28], diet [29], exercise [30], alcohol consumption [28, 31], and ototoxic drug use [32]. Age-related diseases including diabetes [33] and cardiovascular disease [34] are also associated with increased risk of ARHL. Associations between ARHL, environmental and chronic disease factors increase the difficulty of detecting genetic contributions to ARHL, especially as some lifestyle and environmental factors may interact with genetic factors. Accounting for environmental effects could improve the precision of estimates of genetic effects on ARHL, although very large sample sizes are required for analysis of gene-environment interactions. Additionally, in human populations reliable measurement of environmental factors (such as history of work- and leisure-related noise exposure, or recall of use of ototoxic drugs) is challenging.

Despite the challenges of measuring the ARHL phenotype and accounting for NIHL and other environmental impacts on hearing, there are a small but expanding number of studies of the genetics of ARHL. The findings of these studies are grouped according to the possible functional role of the genes in relation to hearing; (1) cell adhesion/cell shape/epithelial development, (2) neurotransmission, (3) oxidative stress, (4) immune response/apoptosis, and (5) other roles.

Studies of the Genetics of ARHL in Humans

Cell Adhesion/Cell Shape/Epithelial Development
Deficits in the structure and/or development of sensory or support cells of the inner ear have been implicated in several types of monogenic hearing loss, so genes related to structure or development are plausible candidates for ARHL (table 1). Van Laer et al. [35] conducted a candidate gene study across 9 centres from 7 European countries with 2,418 participants with audiometric hearing data. A significant association was observed for grainyhead-like 2 (*GRHL2*) variants and hearing. In follow-up analyses, the association was significant in 2 out of the 9 independent subpopulations. *GRHL2* encodes a transcription factor expressed in a variety of epithelial tissues, and is expressed particularly during embryonic development of the cochlea duct.

Table 1. Cell adhesion, cell shape and epithelial development genes associated with ARHL

Gene	Polymorphism	Association	Risk allele	Population	Age, years	Sample size patient/control	Reference
GRHL2	rs10955255 (top hit)	yes[a]	G	Caucasian (European)	53–67	2,418	[35]
	Affymetrix (500K array)	no	–	Caucasian (European)	53–67	1,332	[37]
	Affymetrix (500K array)	no	–	Caucasian (Finnish)	53–67	360	[37]
	rs10955255	no	–	Han Chinese	40–86	310/308	[36]
ITGA8	rs2236579; rs1417664	yes[a]	not given	Caucasian (European)	53–67	2,418	[35]
IQGAP2	rs457717	yes[b]	not given	Finnish Saami	50–75	347	[39]
	rs457717	no	–	Han Chinese (male)	50–100	2,420	[40]
PCDH15	rs7081730 (top hit)	yes[a]	not given	Caucasian (European)	53–67	2,418	[35]
PCDH20	rs78043697 (top hit)	yes[c, d]	C	Italian (isolated population)	18–92	2,155	[38]
		yes[c, d]	C	Silk Road	18–82	481	[38]

GRHL2 = Grainyhead-like 2; ITGA8 = integrin, alpha 8; IQGAP2 = IQ motif containing GTPase activating protein 2; PCDH15 = protocadherin-related 15; PCDH20 = protocadherin 20.
[a] Not significant after Bonferroni correction.
[b] Declared significant at 5×10^{-7}.
[c] Study of normal hearing function.
[d] Significant associations of other SNPs within these genes identified by the same group in cohorts from UK and Finland.

Deficits in *GRHL2* cause a type of monogenic hearing loss (DFNA28). The association between *GRHL2* and ARHL was subsequently not replicated in a Chinese case-control study [36] or in a genome-wide association study (GWAS) with European and Finnish populations [37]. Van Laer et al. [35] reported a further 2 genes involved with epithelial development that showed an association with ARHL. However, the associations did not reach statistical significance after correction for multiple tests. The genes were integrin, alpha 8 (*ITGA8*; implicated in regulation of hair-cell differentiation and stereocilia maturation) and protocadherin-related 15 (*PCDH15*; also implicated in development and maintenance of stereocilia, with mutations in *PCDH15* causing monogenic hearing loss and Usher syndrome type 1).

In a GWAS that included adults aged 18 to 92 years, Vuckovic et al. [38] identified loci for another member of the cadherin superfamily, protocadherin 20 (*PCDH20*; specific function unknown but thought to play a role in the establishment and function of specific cell-cell connections in the brain). The association was replicated in 2 independent cohorts, albeit at a much lower significance value (p = 0.05) and at different audiometric frequencies to those in the discovery sample. Vuckovic et al. [38] reported that *PCDH20* is expressed in the mouse inner ear, supporting a possible functional role for hearing.

Van Laer et al. [39] conducted a GWAS in 347 people from a genetically isolated European population. The use of a genetically isolated population with higher levels of combinations of linked genes in nonrandom proportions (linkage disequilibrium) increased statistical power for a genetic association study. The ARHL phenotype was based on audiometric data classified according to audiogram shape. Van Laer et al. [39] reported a significant association between the 'concavity' of the audiogram and an SNP genetic marker localised in an intron of the IQ motif containing GTPase activating protein 2 (IQGAP2). IQGAP2 encodes a protein that interacts with components of the cytoskeleton, with cadherin-mediated cell adhesion, and with several signalling molecules to regulate cell morphology and motility. IQGAP2 is expressed in the cochlea.

Neurotransmission
Glutamate is the primary excitatory neurotransmitter in the central nervous system. Elevated concentrations of extracellular glutamate cause oxidative stress, excitotoxicity and cell death. Friedman et al. [37] pooling GWAS identified glutamate receptor, metabotropic 7 (GRM7) associated with ARHL. These authors also demonstrated that GRM7 and its protein mGluR7 are found in both hair cells and spiral ganglion cells of the inner ear, and suggested that GRM7 alleles may contribute to the risk of ARHL through altered susceptibility to glutamate excitotoxicity. GRM7 has since been implicated with ARHL by other studies [21, 39, 40], and particular GRM7 variants may occur more frequently with sloping or high frequency losses suggesting involvement with noise-induced and/or sensory hearing loss affecting high frequencies [40] and with measures of peripheral hearing (audiometric threshold and speech reception threshold) rather than measures of temporal or binaural hearing [21] (table 2).

Van Laer et al. [35] observed associations between ARHL and 2 genes for voltage-gated potassium channels, which are functionally related to neuronal excitability (KCNMA1; potassium channel, calcium activated large conductance subfamily M alpha, member 1, and KCNQ1; po-

tassium channel, voltage gated KQT-like subfamily Q, member 1), although associations were not significant after correction for multiple tests. However, Van Eyken et al. [41] reported significant associations between SNPs for KCNQ4 (potassium channel, voltage gated KQT-like subfamily Q, member 4) and ARHL in 2 independent European populations. The protein encoded by KCNQ4 is expressed in hair cells of the cochlea and may play a role in recycling of potassium in the inner ear. Defects in this gene are a cause of an autosomal dominant form of progressive hearing loss (DFNA2). The association between KCNQ4 and ARHL was not replicated by Friedman et al. [37] (table 2).

Finally, in a GWAS of pooled European samples, Vuckovic et al. [38] identified an association between SLC28A3 (solute carrier family 28 (concentrative nucleoside transporter), member 3) and audiometric sensitivity in adults aged 18 to 92 years. SLC28A3 is a nucleoside transporter that regulates multiple cellular processes including neurotransmission. The association was replicated (at a much lower significance value; p = 0.05) in 2 independent cohorts. Follow-up work showed that SLC28A3 is expressed in the mouse inner ear.

Oxidative Stress
Mitochondria are intracellular organelles whose main function is the production of adenosine triphosphate which is the main source of cellular energy. This process generates reactive oxygen species which include hydrogen peroxide, hydroxyl radicals and superoxide anions [42]. The impact of mitochondria on the ageing process and common diseases has been well documented for over half a century, with more recent studies highlighting a complex interaction between mitochondria and other cellular ageing pathways such as those involved in the immune response [43], apoptosis, senescence, and calcium dynamics [44] as well as environmental effects [45]. Eight oxidative stress-related genes have been associated with ARHL

Table 2. Neurotransmission genes associated with ARHL

Gene	Polymorphism	Association	Risk allele	Population	Age, years	Sample size, patient/control	Reference
GRM7	rs11928865	yes	T	Caucasian (European)	53–67	1,332	[37]
	rs11928865	–	–	Caucasian (Finnish)	53–67	360	
	rs779706; rs779701	yes	T	Caucasian (Finnish)	53–67	360	
	rs779706; rs779701	no	–	Caucasian (European)	53–67	1,332	
	rs779701	no	–	Finnish Saami	50–75	347	[39]
	rs161927	yes	A				
	haplotype blocks 6	yes[a]	TT/TT	Caucasian (American)	58 (mean)	687	[21]
	haplotype blocks 7	yes[a]	ATT/ATT				
	rs11928865	yes	T	Han Chinese (male)	71–94	982/324	[40]
KCNMA1	rs697173	yes[b]	not given	Caucasian (European)	53–67	2,418	[35]
KCNQ1	rs12277647	yes[b]	not given	Caucasian (European)	53–67	2,418	[35]
KCNQ4	rs727146	yes[c]	T	Caucasian (Netherlands)	40–80	645	[41]
	rs4660468	yes	not given				
	rs2149034	yes	A				
	rs13374844	yes[c]	not given	Caucasian (Belgium)	55–65	664	[41]
	rs12143503	yes[c]	not given				
	rs727146	yes	not given				
	rs2149034	yes	A				
	Affymetrix (500K array)	no	–	Caucasian (European)	53–67	1,332	[37]
	Affymetrix (500K array)	no	–	Caucasian (Finnish)	53–67	360	
SLC28A3	rs7032430	yes[d]	A	Italian (isolated population)	18–92	2,155	[38]
	rs7032430	yes[d]	A	Silk Road	18–82	481	

GRM7 = Glutamate receptor, metabotropic 7; KCNMA1 = potassium channel, calcium activated large conductance subfamily M alpha, member 1; KCNQ1/KCNQ4 = potassium channel, voltage gated KQT-like subfamily Q, member 1/4; SLC28A3 = solute carrier family 28 (concentrative nucleoside transporter), member 3.
[a] Significant after Bonferroni correction for 2 haplotypes (haplotype block 6: rs11928865, rs9877154 and haplotype block 7: rs3828472, rs9819783, rs11920109).
[b] Not significant after Bonferroni correction.
[c] Sex-genotype interaction observed.
[d] Significant associations of other SNPs within these genes identified by the same group in cohorts from UK and Finland.

(table 3). Of these, *CAT, MTHFR, MTR,* and *UCP2* have yet to be replicated in an independent ARHL cohort. Of the remaining genes (*GSTM1, GSTT1, NAT2,* and *SOD2*) there has been no consistent replication. Below, we give brief details on *GST* and *NAT2* genes which have been studied most extensively.

The glutathione S-transferase genes (*GSTM1* and *GSTT1*) metabolise and detoxify carcinogens, cytotoxins and reactive oxygen species [46]. The initial study by Ates et al. [47] found no association between deletion polymorphisms (where homozygous null individuals produce no protein) in *GSTM1* and *GSTT1* and ARHL using

Table 3. Oxidative stress genes associated with ARHL

Gene	Polymorphism	Association	Risk allele	Population	Age, years	Sample size patient/control	Reference
CAT	rs2300181	yes	not given	Caucasian	53–67	2,418	[35]
GSTM1	GSTM1 null	no	–	Caucasian (Turkish)	61 (mean)	68/69	[47]
	GSTM1 null	yes	deletion	Caucasian (Finnish)	53–67	530	[48]
	GSTM1 null	no	–	Caucasian (European)	53–67	2,010	[48]
	GSTM1 null	yes	deletion	Caucasian	40–81	55/79	[49]
GSTT1	GSTT1 null	no	–	Caucasian (Turkish)	61 (mean)	68/69	[47]
	GSTT1 null	yes[a]	deletion	Caucasian (Finnish)	53–67	530	[48]
	GSTT1 null	no	–	Caucasian (European)	53–67	2,010	[48]
	GSTT1 null	yes	deletion	Caucasian	40–81	55/79	[49]
MTHFR	rs1801133	yes[b]	C	Japanese	40–84	1,426	[73]
MTR	rs1805087	yes[b]	G	Japanese	40–84	1,426	[73]
NAT2	rs1799930 (NAT2*6A)	yes	A	Caucasian (Turkish)	61 (mean)	68/98	[50]
	rs1799930 (NAT2*6A)	yes	A	Caucasian (European)	53–67	2,010	[48]
	rs1799930 (NAT2*6A)	no	–	Caucasian (Finnish)	53–67	530	[48]
	rs1799930 (NAT2*6A)	yes	A	Caucasian	40–81	55/79	[49]
	rs1799930 (NAT2*6A)	no	–	Caucasian (UK)	72 (mean)	265	[51]
	Affymetrix (500K array)	no	–	Caucasian (European)	53–67	1,332	[37]
	Affymetrix (500K array)	no	–	Caucasian (Finnish)	53–67	360	[37]
SOD2	rs5746092	yes[a]	C	Caucasian (London cohort)	NA	585	[67]
	rs5746092	no	–	Caucasian (ELSA cohort)	73 (mean)	529	[67]
UCP2	rs660339 (Ala55Val)	yes	T	Japanese	40–79	1,547	[74]
mtDNA	4,977 deletion	yes	deletion	Chinese	NA	17/17	[75]
	4,977 deletion	yes	deletion	Chinese	NA	34/33	[76]
	all variants	no	–	Caucasian (Belgian)	NA	200/200	[77]

CAT = Catalase; GSTM1 = glutathione S-transferase mu 1; GSTT1 = glutathione S-transferase theta 1; MTHFR = methylenetetrahydrofolate reductase (NAD(P)H); MTR = 5-methyltetrahydrofolate-homocysteine methyltransferase; NAT2 = N-acetyltransferase 2; SOD2 = superoxide dismutase 2, mitochondrial; UCP2 = uncoupling protein 2 (mitochondrial, proton carrier); mtDNA = mitochondrial DNA; ELSA = English longitudinal study of ageing; NA = data not available.
[a] Sex-specific effect.
[b] Epistasis effect.

68 adults with ARHL and 69 healthy controls. An association between these deletions and hearing impairment was observed in a Finnish population (n = 530) but not in a general European population (n = 2,010) [48]. Surprisingly, in the Finnish population those who were homozygous for the GSTM1 deletion had better hearing compared to those without the deletion. In addition, the absence of the GSTT1 deletion was associated with better hearing in the Finnish population but only in women. The most recent study by Bared et al. [49] reported an association between the GSTM1 and GSTT1 deletions in a study of 55 Caucasians with ARHL and 79 controls, in which those with the deletions had worse hearing.

Table 4. Immune/apoptosis genes associated with ARHL

Gene	Polymorphism	Association	Risk allele	Population	Age, years	Sample size	Reference
EYA4	rs212765; rs9321402	yes[a]	not given	Caucasian (European)	53–67	2,418	[35]
TNF	rs1800630	yes	A	Japanese	40–89	1,957	[54]
TNFRSF1B	rs1061624	yes	A	Japanese	40–89	1,957	[54]

EYA4 = EYA transcriptional coactivator and phosphatase 4; *TNF* = tumour necrosis factor; *TNFRSF1B* = tumour necrosis factor receptor superfamily, member 1B.
[a] Not significant after Bonferroni correction.

N-Acetyltransferase 2 *(NAT2)* has been investigated by 5 groups using 7 independent cohorts. The initial study by Ünal et al. [50] found an association between SNP rs1799930 [alias NAT2*6A; G>A (Arg>Gln); missense] in a Turkish population consisting of 68 ARHL patients and 98 controls. In this study, the authors observed a 15.2-fold increased risk in individuals homozygous for the minor allele (A) compared to those homozygous for the wild-type allele (G). A larger independent study, using the Finnish and general European cohorts described above, replicated these findings in the general European cohort but not the Finnish cohort [48]. Further replication of the findings of Ünal et al. was reported by Bared et al. [49] using the Caucasian cohort consisting of 55 patients and 79 controls, which also identified the rs1799930 A allele as the susceptibility allele for ARHL. The most recent attempt at replication using 265 community-dwelling elderly Caucasian individuals failed to find an association between this SNP and ARHL [51] (table 3).

Immune Response/Apoptosis
Ageing is accompanied by increased chronic systemic inflammation, termed 'inflamm-aging' [52], a process which has been associated with hearing loss in community-dwelling elderly [53]. Only 2 groups have reported associations between immune/apoptotic genes and ARHL (table 4). A study of cytokine genes involved in immune homeostasis and the inflammatory response identified SNPs in the tumour necrosis factor gene (*TNF*; rs1800630, located in the proximal promoter region) and tumour necrosis factor receptor superfamily, member 1B gene (*TNFRSF1B*; rs1061624, located in the 3′ untranslated region) that contributed towards hearing impairment in an elderly Japanese population (n = 1,957) [54]. Whilst this study was an investigation of immune response genes, it should be noted that *TNF* is also involved in other processes including apoptosis which itself has also been implicated in ARHL in both animals and humans [55, 56]. Therefore, the mechanism of action of these *TNF* genes, should they be proved to be bona fide susceptibility loci for ARHL, is yet to be determined.

Another gene that has also been implicated in the immune response and apoptosis is EYA transcriptional coactivator and phosphatase 4 *(EYA4)*. This gene encodes a 640-amino-acid transcription factor and has been associated with autosomal dominant nonsyndromic hearing loss [57] and ARHL [35]. In a study of 2,418 ARHL individuals by Van Laer et al. [35], the *EYA4* polymorphism rs212765 was the fourth most significant SNP associated with ARHL from a total of 768 tagging SNPs in 70 candidate genes (the top 3 SNPs were all located in the *GRHL2* gene). Although the association did not remain significant after correction for multiple testing, the previous associations between *EYA4* mutations and other causes of hearing loss make this an interesting candidate gene.

Table 5. Other genes associated with ARHL

Gene	Polymorphism	Association	Risk allele	Population	Age, years	Sample size	Reference
APOE	APOEε4	yes[a]	ε3	NA	34–95	89	[59]
	APOEε2/ε3/ε4	yes[b]	ε4	general population (Leiden)	85	435	[61]
	APOEε4	no	–	Caucasian (UK)	59–88	265	[51]
	APOEε4	yes[a]	ε4	mixed Black/White (USA)	70–79	1,833	[60]
EDN1	rs5370	yes	T	Japanese	40–79	2,231	[78]
ESRRG	rs2818964	yes[c]	A	Caucasian (UK)	44–45	3,900	[63]
	rs2818964	yes[d]	G	Caucasian (London)	71 (mean)	260	
	rs2818964	yes[d]	G	Italian and Silk Road	18–92	1,651	
8q24.13–q24.22	7-Mb region between rs3765212 and rs4601326	yes	–	European descent	49–76	1,126	[17]

APOE = Apolipoprotein E; *EDN1* = endothelin 1; *ESRRG* = estrogen-related receptor gamma; NA = data not available.
[a] APOEε4 associated with better hearing.
[b] APOEε4 associated with worse hearing.
[c] Stronger association observed in males.
[d] Effect observed in females only.

Other Genes

Three other genes *(APOE, EDN1* and *ESRRG)* and a 7-Mb region between 8q24.13 and 8q24.22 have also been associated with ARHL (table 5). Of these, *APOE* and *ESRRG* have been investigated in independent cohorts. *APOE* alleles ε2–4 are the most strongly associated loci for the neurodegenerative condition Alzheimer's disease (www.alzgene.org). Interestingly, *APOE* upregulates N-acetyltransferase expression, suggesting a potential epistasis effect may exist in ARHL [58]. Studies of *APOE* in ARHL have produced inconsistent results. These comprise 2 associations between APOEε4 and better hearing [59, 60]; APOEε4 and worse hearing [61] and no observed association with the ε4 allele [51]. Age differences between these studies may be a factor for these disparate findings with the study using the oldest cohort (85 years of age) reporting the ε4 allele as the susceptibility allele [61]. Indeed, the largest increase in prevalence of ARHL occurs in individuals aged 80 and over [1]. However, by far the largest of these studies (n = 1,833) found that the ε4 allele had a protective effect, albeit a weak one [60].

ARHL has an earlier age of onset and is more severe in men than in women even when noise exposure is adjusted for [62]. Estrogen signalling has been implicated as an auditory protective mechanism and therefore may contribute towards sex-specific effects. Nolan et al. [63] reported that the intronic SNP rs2818964 has been associated with hearing in a study of 3 independent cohorts. In 2 of these cohorts [a cohort of European populations recruited from Italy and Silk Road countries (n = 1,651) and the London ARHL cohort (n = 260)], the effect on hearing was observed in females only with the presence of the minor G allele conferring susceptibility towards hearing loss. In the third cohort (1958 birth cohort), the susceptibility allele was the wild-type A allele, with the association being stronger in males than females. The group further went on to show that *Esrrg* knock-out mice suffered hearing loss at 5 weeks, and by 12 weeks, females had lower hearing thresholds than males.

Future Directions

The genetic field of ARHL is in its infancy compared to genetic studies of other complex genetic diseases and traits such as Alzheimer's disease, schizophrenia, depression, and anthropometric studies such as height and weight. Websites such as Alzgene (www.alzgene.org) and PDgene (www.pdgene.org) list thousands of studies and polymorphisms. In contrast, the genetic study of ARHL has published findings on just over 20 genes with replication (by either an independent group or a second in-house cohort) attempted on just 12 genes. Of these, only *GRM7* has been consistently shown to be associated with ARHL, and the 3 studies that have reported this association have all had a modest sample size.

Genetic association studies of polygenic phenotypes are littered with initial results that fail to replicate. Inadequate sample size, environmental exposure, publication bias, population stratification, and variation in phenotypic classification and measurements are all examples that may make one group's findings different from those of another. As the field of ARHL gains momentum in terms of publication output, it is important to reflect on previous studies of complex diseases and traits in order to help steer research methodologies.

ARHL Phenotype Measurement
The challenge for measurement of the ARHL phenotype involves the need for reliable indices that relate to the underlying pathology of ARHL while being quick and inexpensive enough to use with the very large samples required for genetic studies. Recent applications of internet-based hearing testing that provide a quick, reliable quantitative measure of hearing are promising [18]. Novel screening tests could be validated

against more comprehensive but time-consuming audiometric examinations. Longitudinal measurement that tracks hearing changes over time may be informative in elucidating pathology and defining phenotypes [64].

Sex-Specific Effects
Sex-specific differences in hearing levels have been reported in both longitudinal and cross-sectional studies of ARHL, even in individuals from low-noise occupations who had no evidence of NIHL [62, 65]. These studies have shown that hearing sensitivity declines faster and earlier in men than in women at most frequencies. Of those ARHL genes reported thus far, sex-specific effects have been found for *KCNQ4* [41], *GSTT1* [66], *SOD2*, and *ESRRG* [63, 67]. This may be particularly pertinent for the study of the estrogen receptor *ESRRG* given converging evidence that suggests estrogen is an auditory protectant [63]. Whilst it could be argued that sex-specific analysis may increase the chance of false-positive associations due to multiple testing, the evidence is nevertheless compelling that such differences may be expected, and stratification of males and females should be included when conducting analysis.

Complex Traits Involve Many Loci of Small Effect
All previous GWAS of complex diseases/traits without exception have reported that there are many loci of small effect and that as sample size increases, so too does the number of identified loci [68]. A recent example of this has been observed in 2 studies of educational attainment. The first of these analysed 126,559 individuals and identified 3 SNPs that reached genome-wide significance of 5×10^{-8} or lower [69]. A more recent study applying the same imputation and significance criteria investigated educational attainment using a sample size of 293,723 and identified 74 SNPs, highlighting that as sample size increases so too does the power to detect association. However, even with the considerable power of the latter study, the variance explained by all of the

associated SNPs combined was still <4%. The difference between the expected and observed genetic effect size, termed 'missing heritability', has been observed for all GWAS of complex traits and diseases, and hearing ability is no exception [37–39, 70]. This indicates that either the study of ARHL will require much larger cohorts than have been utilised to date or that researchers need to investigate polymorphisms (such as variable number tandem repeats) or rare mutations which are not currently available on commercial genotyping chips and which may have larger genetic effect sizes compared to currently analysed SNPs. Another explanation for missing heritability may be that combinations of SNPs need to be analysed for the effect to become apparent. Examples of this are the human leukocyte antigen alleles which are a combination of multiple SNPs and the APOEε2–4 alleles which are determined by a combination of 2 SNPs. The high heterogeneity of monogenic hearing loss and the complex nature of ARHL [71] further add to the likelihood that one might expect a very large number of small effect loci to be associated with ARHL.

Conclusion

The genetics of ARHL is a relatively new but rapidly growing area of research with substantial social and economic implications. All studies of complex genetic disorders come with the challenge of avoiding type I and type II errors, and already in ARHL, we are starting to see some inconsistent reports. Whilst using larger sample size replication cohorts and having better defined phenotypes may help alleviate these problems, it is also important to remember that genes are not rigid entities that serve single functions throughout our lives. On the contrary, a single gene may perform multiple tasks, act in tissue- and sex-specific manners, as well as interact with other genes and the environment. The amount of statistical power needed to identify causative variants in ARHL is still unknown, but the recent availability of much larger datasets (including the European G-EAR consortium [70], UK Biobank [72], and the US Million Veteran Program) is likely to shed new light on this exciting area.

References

1 Gates GA, Mills JH: Presbycusis. Lancet 2005;366:1111–1120.
2 Davis AC: The prevalence of hearing impairment and reported hearing disability among adults in Great Britain. Int J Epidemiol 1989;18:911–917.
3 Arlinger S: Negative consequences of uncorrected hearing loss-a review. Int J Audiol 2003;42(suppl 2):2S17–2S20.
4 Shield B: Evaluation of the social and economic costs of hearing impairment. 2006. http://www.hear-it.org/sites/default/files/multimedia/documents/Hear_It_Report_October_2006.pdf.
5 Ruben RJ: Redefining the survival of the fittest: communication disorders in the 21st century. Laryngoscope 2000;110:241–245.
6 Mathers CD, Loncar D: Projections of global mortality and burden of disease from 2002 to 2030. PLoS Med 2006;3:e442.

7 McCormack A, Fortnum H: Why do people fitted with hearing aids not wear them? Int J Audiol 2013;52:360–368.
8 Cruickshanks KJ, Wiley TL, Tweed TS, Klein BE, Klein R, et al: Prevalence of hearing loss in older adults in Beaver Dam, Wisconsin. The Epidemiology of Hearing Loss Study. Am J Epidemiol 1998;148:879–886.
9 Christensen K, Frederiksen H, Hoffman HJ: Genetic and environmental influences on self-reported reduced hearing in the old and oldest old. J Am Geriatr Soc 2001;49:1512–1517.
10 Gates GA, Couropmitree NN, Myers RH: Genetic associations in age-related hearing thresholds. Arch Otolaryngol Head Neck Surg 1999;125:654–659.
11 Karlsoon KK, Harris JR, Svartengren M: Description and primary results from an audiometric study of male twins. Ear Hear 1997;18:114–120.

12 Viljanen A, Era P, Kaprio J, Pyykkö I, Koskenvuo M, Rantanen T: Genetic and environmental influences on hearing in older women. J Gerontol A Biol Sci Med Sci 2007;62:447–452.
13 Schuknecht HF: Further observations on the pathology of presbycusis. Arch Otolaryngol 1964;80:369–382.
14 Schuknecht HF, Gacek MR: Cochlear pathology in presbycusis. Ann Otol Rhinol Laryngol 1993;102:1–16.
15 Allen PD, Eddins DA: Presbycusis phenotypes form a heterogeneous continuum when ordered by degree and configuration of hearing loss. Hear Res 2010;264:10–20.
16 Scholtz AW, Kammen-Jolly K, Felder E, Hussl B, Rask-Andersen H, Schrott-Fischer A: Selective aspects of human pathology in high-tone hearing loss of the aging inner ear. Hear Res 2001;157:77–86.

17 Huyghe JR, Van Laer L, Hendrickx JJ, Fransen E, Demeester K, et al: Genome-wide SNP-based linkage scan identifies a locus on 8q24 for an age-related hearing impairment trait. Am J Hum Genet 2008;83:401–407.

18 Wolber LE, Steves CJ, Spector TD, Williams FM: Hearing ability with age in Northern European women: a new web-based approach to genetic studies. PLoS One 2012;7:e35500.

19 Wolber LE, Girotto G, Buniello A, Vuckovic D, Pirastu N, et al: Salt-inducible kinase 3, SIK3, is a new gene associated with hearing. Hum Mol Genet 2014;23:6407–6418.

20 Momi SK, Wolber LE, Fabiane SM, MacGregor AJ, Williams FM: Genetic and environmental factors in age-related hearing impairment. Twin Res Hum Genet 2015;18:383–392.

21 Newman DL, Fisher LM, Ohmen J, Parody R, Fong CT, et al: GRM7 variants associated with age-related hearing loss based on auditory perception. Hear Res 2012;294:125–132.

22 Yamasoba T, Lin FR, Someya S, Kashio A, Sakamoto T, Kondo K: Current concepts in age-related hearing loss: epidemiology and mechanistic pathways. Hear Res 2013;303:30–38.

23 Jiang H, Talaska AE, Schacht J, Sha SH: Oxidative imbalance in the aging inner ear. Neurobiol Aging 2007;28:1605–1612.

24 Ohlemiller KK: Mechanisms and genes in human strial presbycusis from animal models. Brain Res 2009;1277:70–83.

25 ACOEM Noise and Hearing Conservation Committee: ACOEM evidence-based statement: noise-induced hearing loss. J Occup Environ Med 2003;45:579–581.

26 Gong TW, Lomax MI: Genes that influence susceptibility to noise-induced hearing loss; in Le Prell CG, Henderson D, Fay RR, Popper AN (eds): Noise-Induced Hearing Loss. New York, Springer, 2012, pp 179–203.

27 Nomura K, Nakao M, Morimoto T: Effect of smoking on hearing loss: quality assessment and meta-analysis. Prev Med 2005;40:138–144.

28 Dawes P, Cruickshanks KJ, Moore DR, Edmondson-Jones M, McCormack A, et al: Cigarette smoking, passive smoking, alcohol consumption and hearing loss. J Assoc Res Otolaryngol 2014;15:663–674.

29 Spankovich C: The role of nutrition in healthy hearing: human evidence; in Miller J, le Prell CG, Rybak L (eds): Free Radicals in ENT Pathology. New York, Humana Press, 2015, pp 111–126.

30 Hull RH, Kerschen SR: The influence of cardiovascular health on peripheral and central auditory function in adults: a research review. Am J Audiol 2010;19:9–16.

31 Popelka MM, Cruickshanks KJ, Wiley TL, Tweed TS, Klein BE, et al: Moderate alcohol consumption and hearing loss: a protective effect. J Am Geriatr Soc 2000;48:1273–1278.

32 Scott PMJ, Griffiths MV: A clinical review of ototoxicity. Clin Otolaryngol Allied Sci 1994;19:3–8.

33 Horikawa C, Kodama S, Tanaka S, Fujihara K, Hirasawa R, et al: Diabetes and risk of hearing impairment in adults: a meta-analysis. J Clin Endocrinol Metab 2013;98:51–58.

34 Helzner EP, Patel AS, Pratt S, Sutton-Tyrrell K, Cauley JA, et al: Hearing sensitivity in older adults: associations with cardiovascular risk factors in the health, aging and body composition study. J Am Geriatr Soc 2011;59:972–979.

35 Van Laer L, Van Eyken E, Fransen E, Huyghe JR, Topsakal V, et al: The grainyhead like 2 gene (GRHL2), alias TFCP2L3, is associated with age-related hearing impairment. Hum Mol Genet 2008;17:159–169.

36 Lin YH, Wu CC, Hsu CJ, Hwang JH, Liu TC: The grainyhead-like 2 gene (GRHL2) single nucleotide polymorphism is not associated with age-related hearing impairment in Han Chinese. Laryngoscope 2011;121:1303–1307.

37 Friedman RA, Van Laer L, Huentelman MJ, Sheth SS, Van Eyken E, et al: GRM7 variants confer susceptibility to age-related hearing impairment. Hum Mol Genet 2009;18:785–796.

38 Vuckovic D, Dawson S, Scheffer DI, Rantanen T, Morgan A, et al: Genome-wide association analysis on normal hearing function identifies PCDH20 and SLC28A3 as candidates for hearing function and loss. Hum Mol Genet 2015;24:5655–5664.

39 Van Laer L, Huyghe JR, Hannula S, Van Eyken E, Stephan DA, et al: A genome-wide association study for age-related hearing impairment in the Saami. Eur J Hum Genet 2010;18:685–693.

40 Luo H, Yang T, Jin X, Pang X, Li J, et al: Association of GRM7 variants with different phenotype patterns of age-related hearing impairment in an elderly male Han Chinese population. PLoS One 2013;8:e77153.

41 Van Eyken E, Van Laer L, Fransen E, Topsakal V, Lemkens N, et al: KCNQ4: a gene for age-related hearing impairment? Hum Mutat 2006;27:1007–1016.

42 Balaban RS, Nemoto S, Finkel T: Mitochondria, oxidants, and aging. Cell 2005;120:483–495.

43 De la Fuente M, Miquel J: An update of the oxidation-inflammation theory of aging: the involvement of the immune system in oxi-inflamm-aging. Curr Pharm Des 2009;15:3003–3026.

44 Gonzalez-Freire M, de Cabo R, Bernier M, Sollott SJ, Fabbri E, et al: Reconsidering the role of mitochondria in aging. J Gerontol A Biol Sci Med Sci 2015;70:1334–1342.

45 Payne BA, Chinnery PF: Mitochondrial dysfunction in aging: much progress but many unresolved questions. Biochim Biophys Acta 2015;1847:1347–1353.

46 Beckett GJ, Hayes JD: Glutathione S-transferases: biomedical applications. Adv Clin Chem 1993;30:281–380.

47 Ates NA, Unal M, Tamer L, Derici E, Karakaş S, et al: Glutathione S-transferase gene polymorphisms in presbycusis. Otol Neurotol 2005;26:392–397.

48 Van Eyken E, Van Camp G, Fransen E, Topsakal V, Hendrickx JJ, et al: Contribution of the N-acetyltransferase 2 polymorphism NAT2*6A to age-related hearing impairment. J Med Genet 2007;44:570–578.

49 Bared A, Ouyang X, Angeli S, Du LL, Hoang K, et al: Antioxidant enzymes, presbycusis, and ethnic variability. Otolaryngol Head Neck Surg 2010;143:263–268.

50 Ünal M, Tamer L, Doğruer ZN, Yildirim H, Vayisoğlu Y, Camdeviren H: N-acetyltransferase 2 gene polymorphism and presbycusis. Laryngoscope 2005;115:2238–2241.

51 Dawes P, Platt H, Horan M, Ollier W, Munro K, et al: No association between apolipoprotein E or N-acetyltransferase 2 gene polymorphisms and age-related hearing loss. Laryngoscope 2015;125:E33–E38.

52 Franceschi C, Bonafè M, Valensin S, Olivieri F, De Luca M, et al: Inflammaging. An evolutionary perspective on immunosenescence. Ann N Y Acad Sci 2000;908:244–254.

53 Verschuur CA, Dowell A, Syddall HE, Ntani G, Simmonds SJ, et al: Markers of inflammatory status are associated with hearing threshold in older people: findings from the Hertfordshire Ageing Study. Age Ageing 2012;41:92–97.

54 Uchida Y, Sugiura S, Ueda H, Nakashima T, Ando F, Shimokata H: The association between hearing impairment and polymorphisms of genes encoding inflammatory mediators in Japanese aged population. Immun Ageing 2014; 11:18.

55 Xiong H, Pang J, Yang H, Dai M, Liu Y, Ou Y, et al: Activation of miR-34a/SIRT1/p53 signaling contributes to cochlear hair cell apoptosis: implications for age-related hearing loss. Neurobiol Aging 2015;36:1692–1701.

56 Dong Y, Li M, Liu P, Song H, Zhao Y, Shi J: Genes involved in immunity and apoptosis are associated with human presbycusis based on microarray analysis. Acta Otolaryngol 2014;134:601–608.

57 Kim Y, Kim MA, Sagong B, Bae SH, Lee HJ, et al: Evaluation of the contribution of the EYA4 and GRHL2 genes in Korean patients with autosomal dominant non-syndromic hearing loss. PLoS One 2015;10:e0119443.

58 Liu Y, Meng FT, Wang LL, Zhang LF, Cheng XP, Zhou JN: Apolipoprotein E influences melatonin biosynthesis by regulating NAT and MAOA expression in C6 cells. J Pineal Res 2012;52:397–402.

59 O'Grady G, Boyles AL, Speer M, DeRuyter F, Strittmatter W, Worley G: Apolipoprotein E alleles and sensorineural hearing loss. Int J Audiol 2007;46:183–186.

60 Mener DJ, Betz J, Yaffe K, Harris TB, Helzner EP, et al: Apolipoprotein E allele and hearing thresholds in older adults. Am J Alzheimers Dis Other Demen 2016;31:34–39.

61 Kurniawan C, Westendorp RG, de Craen AJ, Gussekloo J, de Laat J, van Exel E: Gene dose of apolipoprotein E and age-related hearing loss. Neurobiol Aging 2012;33:2230.e7–e12.

62 Pearson JD, Morrell CH, Gordon-Salant S, Brant LJ, Metter EJ, et al: Gender differences in a longitudinal study of age-associated hearing loss. J Acoust Soc Am 1995;97:1196–1205.

63 Nolan LS, Maier H, Hermans-Borgmeyer I, Girotto G, Ecob R, et al: Estrogen-related receptor gamma and hearing function: evidence of a role in humans and mice. Neurobiol Aging 2013;34:2077.e1–e9.

64 Gates GA, Schmid P, Kujawa SG, Nam B, D'Agostino R: Longitudinal threshold changes in older men with audiometric notches. Hear Res 2000;141:220–228.

65 Blanchet C, Pommie C, Mondain M, Berr C, Hillaire D, Puel JL: Pure-tone threshold description of an elderly French screened population. Otol Neurotol 2008;29:432–440.

66 Van Eyken E, Van Camp G, Van Laer L: The complexity of age-related hearing impairment: contributing environmental and genetic factors. Audiol Neurotol 2007;12:345–358.

67 Nolan LS, Cadge BA, Gomez-Dorado M, Dawson SJ: A functional and genetic analysis of SOD2 promoter variants and their contribution to age-related hearing loss. Mech Ageing Dev 2013;134:298–306.

68 Visscher PM, Brown MA, McCarthy MI, Yang J: Five years of GWAS discovery. Am J Hum Genet 2012;90:7–24.

69 Rietveld CA, Medland SE, Derringer J, Yang J, Esko T, et al: GWAS of 126,559 individuals identifies genetic variants associated with educational attainment. Science 2013;340:1467–1471.

70 Girotto G, Pirastu N, Sorice R, Biino G, Campbell H, et al: Hearing function and thresholds: a genome-wide association study in European isolated populations identifies new loci and pathways. J Med Genet 2011;48:369–374.

71 Kubisch C: Hereditary hearing loss in humans: the importance of genetic approaches for clinical medicine and basic science. e-Neuroforum 2014;5:67–71.

72 Collins R: What makes UK Biobank special? Lancet 2012;379:1173–1174.

73 Uchida Y, Sugiura S, Ando F, Nakashima T, Shimokata H: Hearing impairment risk and interaction of folate metabolism related gene polymorphisms in an aging study. BMC Med Genet 2011; 12:35.

74 Sugiura S, Uchida Y, Nakashima T, Ando F, Shimokata H: The association between gene polymorphisms in uncoupling proteins and hearing impairment in Japanese elderly. Acta Otolaryngol 2010;130:487–492.

75 Bai U, Seidman MD, Hinojosa R, Quirk WS: Mitochondrial DNA deletions associated with aging and possibly presbycusis: a human archival temporal bone study. Am J Otol 1997;18:449–453.

76 Dai P, Yang W, Jiang S, Gu R, Yuan H, et al: Correlation of cochlear blood supply with mitochondrial DNA common deletion in presbyacusis. Acta Otolaryngol 2004;124:130–136.

77 Bonneux S, Fransen E, Van Eyken E, Van Laer L, Huyghe J, et al: Inherited mitochondrial variants are not a major cause of age-related hearing impairment in the European population. Mitochondrion 2011;11:729–734.

78 Uchida Y, Sugiura S, Nakashima T, Ando F, Shimokata H: Endothelin-1 gene polymorphism and hearing impairment in elderly Japanese. Laryngoscope 2009;119:938–943.

Piers Dawes, PhD
School of Psychological Sciences
The University of Manchester, Ellen Wilkinson Building
Oxford Road, Manchester M13 9PL (UK)
E-Mail piers.dawes@manchester.ac.uk

Vona B, Haaf T (eds): Genetics of Deafness. Monogr Hum Genet. Basel, Karger, 2016, vol 20, pp 97–109
(DOI: 10.1159/000444568)

Genetic Modifiers of Hearing Loss in Mice: The Case of Phenotypic Modification in Homozygous *Cdh23ahl* Age-Related Hearing Loss

Yoshiaki Kikkawa · Yuki Miyasaka

Mammalian Genetics Project, Department of Genome Medicine, Tokyo Metropolitan Institute of Medical Science, Tokyo, and Graduate School of Medical and Dental Sciences, Niigata University, Niigata, Japan

Abstract

There has been considerable progress in identifying the mutations primarily associated with congenital hearing loss caused by a single gene. The next challenge is the discovery of genes and mutations associated with common acquired hearing loss in the human population such as age-related hearing loss (AHL) and presbyacusis, which occur through the effects of environmental risk factors and several quantitative trait loci, namely, genetic modifiers. One approach to identify novel modifier genes is an unbiased genomic strategy that utilizes mouse models, which are investigated in a controlled environment. Here, we describe the genetic modifiers that contribute to hearing loss susceptibility and resistance in inbred mice and the genetic approaches used to identify the modifiers in the genetic background, with emphasis on the AHL mutation of the cadherin 23 gene *Cdh23ahl*. *Cdh23ahl* is the mutation responsible for hearing loss in multiple inbred strains and impacts mice hearing phenotypes as a genetic modifier. We then discuss the AHL-resistance effect in the presence of *Cdh23ahl* identified using a chromosomal substitution (consomic) strain. Finally, we propose future directions for identifying genetic modifiers using forward and reverse genetics approaches.

© 2016 S. Karger AG, Basel

Genetic modifiers are an integral part of the genetic landscape of human disease [1]. In hearing loss, the identification and functional analysis of genetic modifiers provides considerable knowledge on the phenotypic heterogeneity of Mendelian disorders and the genetic pathways and networks through genetic and molecular analyses of susceptibility and resistance modulation by mutant phenotypes in genetic hearing loss. However, most effects of genetic modifiers for hearing loss on human phenotypes are less understood because the identification of genetic modifiers has commonly been used for quantitative trait locus

(QTL) mapping [1], which is difficult in human populations compromised by sample size of the family, genetic divergence of individuals, and the influence of environmental modifiers, such as exposure to noise, ototoxic drugs, viral and bacterial infections, disease complications, and aging [2]. In particular, due to the influence of these environmental modifiers with aging, the difficulty in identifying genetic modifiers is greater for acquired hearing loss disorders, such as progressive hearing loss, age-related hearing loss (AHL) and presbyacusis.

To identify genetic modifiers associated with acquired hearing loss, as a complementary approach to human study, the mouse is a useful bioresource because it can be investigated in a controlled environment. Moreover, mice are maintained with stable genetic backgrounds [3, 4], and the genetic diversity among inbred strains is well characterized [5, 6]. Inbred strains offer important advantages for identifying modifiers associated with AHL because many AHL susceptibility and resistance strains have been characterized through phenotypic hearing analyses [3, 4, 7]. Through QTL linkage mapping studies using backcrossing and F_2 progeny, recombinant inbred (RI) strains and chromosomal substitution (consomic) strains established from AHL susceptibility and resistance strains, a growing number of loci and mutations of genes that modify AHL have been successfully identified in mice [reviewed in 3, 4].

This chapter applied the advantages of mouse genetics to the study of genetic modifiers of hearing. This article will discuss AHL modification by the *ahl* mutation of the cadherin 23 gene *Cdh23^{ahl}*. *Cdh23^{ahl}* is responsible for AHL in multiple inbred mouse strains [8], and the AHL phenotypes are modulated by epistatic (interactive) and additive (multiplicative) effects between *Cdh23^{ahl}* and its modifiers. These findings are informative and interesting examples to introduce and explain the advantages of mouse models in the analysis of genetic modifiers.

Tip Link Protein Cadherin 23

Cadherin 23 (CDH23), known as otocadherin, is a member of the cadherin superfamily of cell surface adhesion proteins containing 27 extracellular (EC) cadherin repeats, followed by a single transmembrane domain and a short intracellular domain (fig. 1a) [9–11]. The association of *Cdh23* mutations with hearing loss was first identified in waltzer *Cdh23^v* mutant mice [9] and humans with type I Usher syndrome (USH1) [10]. USH1 is a severe disorder that causes profound congenital hearing loss, along with vestibular dysfunction and vision loss beginning in childhood [10, 11]. Functionally null *Cdh23^v* mutants exhibit typical shaker/waltzer behaviors, such as circling, head tossing and hyperactivity, together with profound congenital hearing loss, which is caused by disorganization of the stereocilia in the inner ear hair cells [9]. Figure 1b shows the 'V'-shaped and staircase-like architecture of mature stereocilia in the outer hair cell (OHC) of the cochlea. CDH23 protein is localized at the tip link (fig. 1c) [12], connecting shorter stereocilia to the shafts of the adjacent taller stereocilia (fig. 1b, d) and gating the mechanoelectrical transduction channels that convey mechanical forces, such as sound and gravity [13]. The tip links are formed by a tetramer of CDH23 and another cadherin, protocadherin 15 (PCDH15) (fig. 1d) [11, 13–15], which is also responsible for human USH1 and mouse Ames waltzer mutants *Pcdh15^{av}*, which exhibit a similar phenotype as *Cdh23^v* mice [16, 17]. CDH23 and PCDH15 are also expressed in developing bundles, where they localize to transient lateral and kinocilial links [18, 19]; the interaction between the 2 cadherins is important for maintaining the morphology and cohesion of the bundles through the tension of the stereocilial links. Moreover, the function of CDH23 and PCDH15 is suggested by the degeneration of stereocilia in mutant mice lacking both cadherins, which is caused by the disruption of bundle cohesion during stereocilia development.

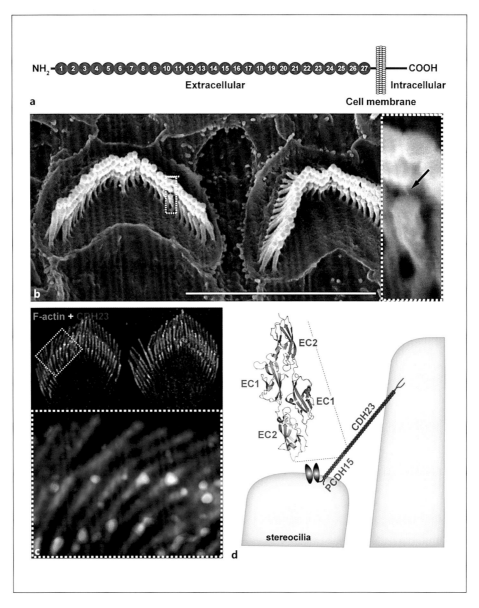

Fig. 1. CDH23 protein is a component of the tip link. **a** Schematic diagram of the CDH23 protein structure. Gray circles indicate EC cadherin repeats. **b** Scanning electron microscope image of OHC in mouse. The right panel shows a highly magnified image of the dashed box in the left panel. The arrow indicates a tip link connecting a shorter stereocilium to the shaft of the adjacent taller stereocilium. Scale bar = 5 μm. **c** High-resolution immunohistochemical image of CDH23 (red) in OHCs using stimulated emission depletion (STED) microscopy. Stereocilia are visualized by phalloidin staining (green). The bottom panel shows a highly magnified image of the dashed box in the top panel. **d** Schematic illustrating a tip link formed by an interaction between a parallel dimer of CDH23 (red) and PCDH15 (blue). A ribbon diagram (PDB ID: 4AXW) [15] illustrates binding in the EC1 and EC2 domains of both otocadherins.

Effect of Cdh23*ahl* Allele Homozygosity on AHL

Additionally, *Cdh23* mutation is responsible for AHL in mice. The susceptibility locus for AHL is designated *ahl* and was mapped to chromosome 10 by genetic analysis using crosses of AHL-susceptible C57BL/6J and AHL-resistant CAST/Ei strains [20]. Subsequently, the responsible *Cdh23*^ahl^ mutation (c.753G>A) was identified at the last position of exon 7 of *Cdh23*, one base before the splice-donor site, causing skipping of exon 7 and leading to an in-frame deletion of 43 amino acids comprising part of the EC2–3 domain of CDH23 protein (fig. 2a, b) [8]. Although the hearing levels detected by measuring of auditory brainstem response (ABR) differed between research groups due to the differences in conditions such as auditory stimulations and instruments for measurements, C57BL/6J mice, which possess a homozygous *Cdh23*^ahl^ mutation, develop severe AHL without exception at the older age (table 1) [7, 21–24]. The AHL of C57BL/6J mice may be associated with age-related stereocilia degeneration in cochlear hair cells. Although the development of the stereocilia bundles is unaffected in C57BL/6J mice, stereocilia become degenerated at older ages (fig. 2c) [23]. Another hypomorphic mutation of *Cdh23*, *Cdh23*^salsa^, causes progressive loss of the tip links in mice [25]. These findings suggest that CDH23 contributes not only to the development of stereocilia but also to the maintenance of stereocilia and tip links. In addition, C57BL/6J mice display loss of spiral ganglion cells (SGCs) with aging (fig. 2c) [20, 26]. Oxidative damage (reactive oxygen species, ROS) leads to the loss of spiral ganglion neurons and sensory hair cells in the ear during aging, resulting in age-related hearing loss [26, 27]. Therefore, SGC degeneration in C57BL/6J mice may indicate that weakened and broken tip links due to *Cdh23*^ahl^ mutation homozygosity are more susceptible to ROS, leading to oxidative stress-induced apoptosis of hair cells and SGCs during aging.

Epistatic and Additive Effects between Cdh23*ahl* and Other Modifiers in the Hearing Loss of Inbred Mouse Strains

Noben-Trauth et al. [8] reported that the *Cdh23*^753A^ mutation is an inbred strain-specific dimorphism in multiple inbred mouse strains. Table 1 shows inbred strains carrying the *Cdh23*^ahl^ mutation listed in the JAX Mouse Database (The Jackson Laboratory, http://www.jax.org/index. html) and the age (in weeks) at which the ABR threshold (<71 dB SPL) of severe hearing loss is reached in their strains, as reported by several groups. The onset of severe hearing loss has been recognized in 17 inbred strains carrying the *Cdh23*^ahl^ mutation. Interestingly, the *Cdh23*^ahl^ homozygous inbred strains are classified into groups of early-onset and late-onset hearing loss (table 1). The early-onset hearing loss group has additional susceptibility modifiers in their genetic background, and the age of onset and severity of hearing loss may be accelerated by epistatic and additive effects between *Cdh23*^ahl^ and modifiers. Indeed, the A/J [28], BUB/BnJ [29], DBA/2J [30], and NOD/ShiLtJ [31] strains develop early-onset hearing loss only with homozygosity of the *Cdh23*^ahl^ allele using QTL linkage analyses (table 1).

A typical example of epistatic effects with *Cdh23*^ahl^ is the early-onset hearing loss in DBA/2J mice. Hearing loss in DBA/2J mice rapidly progresses to the low frequencies from ultrasonic frequencies and to levels of severe hearing loss at 4–28 weeks of age (table 1) [7, 24, 30, 32]. Johnson et al. [30] found that the *ahl8* locus is linked to the early-onset hearing loss of DBA/2J mice using genetic analyses on BXD RI strains and (C57BL/6J × DBA/2J) × DBA/2J backcrossed mice. Moreover, this study confirmed that *Cdh23*^ahl^ greatly contributes to early-onset hearing loss in DBA/2J mice by investigating the association between ABR thresholds and genotypes of *Cdh23*^ahl^ and *ahl8* locus in (B6. CAST-*Cdh23*^Ahl+^ congenic × DBA/2J) × DBA/2J backcrossed mice. Subsequently, the responsible

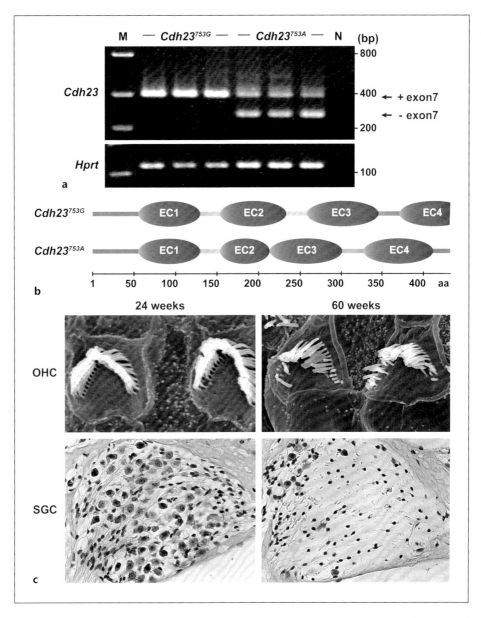

Fig. 2. The *Cdh23^ahl* mutation is responsible for hair cell and SGC degeneration in the organ of Corti in aging mice. **a** Partial alternatively spliced products revealed through the *Cdh23^ahl* (c.753G>A) mutation. The upper panel shows the electrophoretic profile of RT-PCR products amplified from cochlear cDNA from *Cdh23^753A* and *Cdh23^753G* homozygous mice using *Cdh23*-specific primers located in exons 6 and 8 [23]. The 396 bp (+ exon 7) and 267 bp (– exon 7) bands are presented by *Cdh23^753A* homozygous mice. cDNA integrity was confirmed using a hypoxanthine-guanine phosphoribosyl transferase *Hprt* control band (bottom panel). M = Marker (DNA ladder); N = negative control. **b** Schematic diagrams of the domain architectures (EC1–4) of CDH23 encoded from *Cdh23^753G* (top) and *Cdh23^753A* (bottom) alleles predicted by the SMART program (http://smart.embl-heidelberg.de/). **c** Morphological comparison of OHCs (top) and SGCs (bottom) in C57BL/6J mice at 24 weeks (left) and 60 weeks (right) of age.

Table 1. Inbred mouse strains carrying homozygous $Cdh23^{ahl/ahl}$ alleles and the onset age of severe hearing loss

Strain	Weeks of age ABR thresholds were measured	Auditory stimulation	Weeks of age at which severe hearing loss developed (71–90 dB SPL)			Reference
			8 kHz	16 kHz	32 kHz	
129P1/ReJ	9, 13, 28	tone burst	ND	28	28	[7]
129P3/J	9, 12, 23	tone burst	23	23	12	[7]
129X1/SvJ	9, 13, 45	tone burst	45	45	45	[7]
A/J	8, 10, 13, 30	tone burst	ND	30	30	[7]
	3–4, 8, 24	tone burst	8	8	3–4	[28]
A/WySnJ	8, 34	tone burst	ND	ND	ND	[7]
ALR/LtJ	40	tone burst	40	40	40	[7]
	5	tone pip	5	5	5	[60]
ALS/LtJ	26	tone burst	26	26	26	[7]
BALB/cByJ	34	tone burst	ND	ND	ND	[7]
BUB/BnJ	3, 8, 13, 20	tone burst	8	6	6	[7]
	3, 8–13, 20	tone burst	8–13	8–13	3	[29]
C57BL/6J	27, 33, 100	tone burst	100	100	100	[7]
	12, 24, 36, 48, 60, 48	tone burst	60	72	24	[21]
	4–8, 9, 12, 15, 18, 21, 24	tone pip	21	21	24	[22]
	4–48 at 4-week intervals	tone pip	ND	40	20	[23]
	12	tone pip	ND	ND	12	[24]
C57BLKS/J	11, 15, 45	tone burst	ND	45	45	[7]
C57BR/cdJ	7, 20, 34, 68	tone burst	34	ND	20	[7]
C57L/J	9, 32, 42, 50, 70	tone burst	9	ND	9	[7]
C58/J	9, 30	tone burst	ND	ND	30	[7]
CE/J	12, 50	tone burst	ND	ND	ND	[7]
DBA/1J	48	tone burst	ND	ND	ND	[7]
DBA/1LacJ	33	tone burst	ND	33	33	[7]
DBA/2J	3, 5, 8, 11, 14, 28, 44	tone burst	28	28	11	[7]
	12	tone pip	12	12	12	[24]
	3–4, 10, 27	tone burst	27	10	10	[30]
	4–48 at 4-week intervals	tone pip	16	4	4	[32]
KK/HlJ	8, 50	tone burst	ND	ND	ND	[7]
LG/J	8, 28, 48	tone burst	ND	ND	ND	[7]
LP/J	11, 31, 49	tone burst	ND	ND	ND	[7]
MA/MyJ	6, 13, 48	tone burst	48	48	48	[7]
NOD/ShiLtJ	3, 5, 8, 11, 14, 28, 44	tone burst	28	28	11	[7]
NOR/LtJ	9, 15, 34	tone burst	9	9	9	[7]
P/J	10, 16, 19	tone burst	ND	ND	ND	[7]
SENCARB/PtJ	39	tone burst	ND	ND	ND	[7]

ND = Not determined.

$Fscn2^{ahl8}$ mutation (p.109Arg>His) was observed in the fascin 2 gene $Fscn2$, encoding an actin crosslinking protein (table 2) [33]. DBA/2J mice display progressive shortening of rows 2 and 3 of the stereocilia bundles, and the phenotype only presents with homozygosity of both the $Cdh23^{ahl}$ and $Fscn2^{ahl8}$ alleles [33, 34]. FSCN2 protein localizes along the length of stereocilia, with high concentration around the stereocilial tip [33, 34]. Biochemical analysis indicates that

Table 2. Modification of hearing loss in mice by epistatic and additive effects between $Cdh23^{ahl/ahl}$ homozygosity and other loci (mutations)

Strain	Locus/gene symbol	Chr	Causative mutation	Reference
Inbred strain				
A/J	Cs^{ahl4}	10	p.55His>Asn	[28, 43]
	$mt\text{-}Tr^{Arg}$	mtDNA	single adenine insertion	[42]
BUB/BnJ	$Gpr98^{frings}$	13	p.2072Val>X	[29]
DBA/2J	$Fscn2^{ahl8}$	11	p.109Arg>His	[30, 33, 34]
MSM/Ms	$ahl3$	17	unknown	[52, 54]
NOD/ShiLtJ	$ahl2$	5	unknown	[31]
Mutant strain				
$Actb^{flox/flox}$, $Atoh1\text{-}cre$ cKO	$Actb$	5	KO	[34]
$Sod1^{-/-}$ KO	$Sod1$	16	KO	[51]
$Atp2b2^{dfw/+}$ heterozygotes	$Atp2b2^{dfw\text{-}2J,\ dfw\text{-}i5}$	6	p.457GlyfsX15, p.580Lys>X	[48, 49]

$Actb$ = Actin, beta; ahl = age-related hearing loss; $Atp2b2$ = ATPase, Ca^{2+} transporting, plasma membrane 2; Chr = chromosome; cKO = conditional KO; cre = Cre recombinase; Cs = citrate synthase; dfw = deafwaddler; $flox$ = floxed; $Fscn2$ = fascin 2; $Gpr98$ = G protein-coupled receptor 98; KO = knockout; $mt\text{-}Tr^{Arg}$ = mitochondrial arginine tRNA; $Sod1$ = superoxide dismutase 1, soluble.

the $Fscn2^{ahl8}$ mutation prevents efficient actin crosslinking [34]. Although the detailed molecular mechanisms in the genetic interaction between CDH23 and FSCN2 remain unknown, these findings suggest that both proteins contribute to the length regulation of stereocilia at the tip link. Moreover, frequency-specific QTLs contributing to early-onset hearing loss have been mapped onto chromosomes 5 [32] and 18 [24] in DBA/2J mice, suggesting that DBA/2J mice represent a typical model for frequency-specific hearing loss according to the contributions of different QTLs. In addition, BUB/BnJ mice may also develop hearing loss through epistatic effects. Although BUB/BnJ mice display audiogenic seizures [35] caused by the frings $Adgrv1^{frings}$ mutation (table 2) of the adhesion G protein-coupled receptor V1 gene $Adgrv1$, also known as $Mass1$, $Vlgr1$ and $Gpr98$, the mice develop severe early-onset hearing loss by 3–13 weeks of age (table 1) [7, 29]. Johnson et al. [29] reported that the progression of hearing loss in BUB/BnJ mice is moderated by homozygosity of

$Cdh23^{ahl}$. The ADGRV1 protein is a member of the adhesion receptor family within the 7 transmembrane receptor superfamily and is responsible for type II Usher syndrome (USH2) [36]. In hair cells, ADGRV1 is transiently localized in the transient ankle links of stereocilia [37, 38]. Moreover, Zallocchi et al. [39, 40] indicated that ADGRV1 is also expressed at the ribbon synapses of hair cells and forms a complex with Clarin-1, CDH23, and PCDH15.

In contrast, we predict that the A/J mouse strain is a model of hearing loss modulation via additive effects of the $Cdh23^{ahl}$ mutation and other genetic modifiers. A/J mice develop early-onset hearing loss prior to 30 weeks of age (table 1) [7, 28], which is associated with OHC and SGC loss [41]. The significant linkage of AHL with A/J mice and $Cdh23^{ahl}$ was confirmed by an association study using (A/J × CAST/Ei) F_1 × A/J backcrossed mice [42]. This study also reported that mitochondrial DNA (mtDNA) derived from the A/J strain enhances hearing loss compared with that of CAST/Ei and carries a single adenine insertion in the mitochondrial tRNA-Arg gene $mt\text{-}Tr^{Arg}$ (table 2). Moreover, the *ahl4* susceptibility locus and the responsible Cs^{ahl4} mutation (p.55His>Asn) of citrate synthase *Cs* were identified via genotype-phenotype associations of the AXB and BXA RI, C57BL/6J-Chr 10$^{A/J}$/NaJ consomic, and C57BL/6J-Chr 10$^{A/J}$ congenic strains (table 2) [28, 43]. CS protein is a rate-limiting enzyme of the tricarboxylic acid cycle that plays a decisive role in regulating energy generation through mitochondrial respiration [44]. Several reports have indicated that mutations of the mtDNA genome lead to hearing loss in human populations [45]. ROS generated inside mitochondria are hypothesized to damage mitochondrial components, mtDNA, mitochondrial membranes, and respiration-related proteins such as CS [26, 46]. Moreover, Han et al. [41] suggested that reduction of CS activity leads to caspase-mediated apoptosis in type II-like cells of an inner ear cell line and A/J mice in in vitro and in vivo experiments, respectively. These findings may indicate that the early-onset hearing loss of A/J mice is accelerated by death of OHCs and SGCs, causing excess ROS generation, which leads to mitochondrial dysfunction via the Cs^{ahl4} and $mt\text{-}Tr^{Arg}$ mutations. Thus, the $Cdh23^{ahl}$ tip link component mutation and mitochondrial-related mutations constitute different underlying pathological mechanisms in the inner ear, suggesting that A/J mice develop early-onset hearing loss from additive effects of different functional mutations.

Phenotypic Modification of the $Cdh23^{ahl}$ Allele in Hearing Loss of Deaf Mutant Mice

The $Cdh23^{ahl}$ mutation is the most common modifier for hearing loss in mice (table 2). The typical example is modification of the onset of hearing loss in heterozygous deaf waddler $Atp2b2^{dfw}$ mutant mice affected in the plasma membrane calcium (Ca^{2+}) ATPase 2 gene $Atp2b2$. $Atp2b2^{dfw/dfw}$ homozygous mice exhibit

profound and congenital hearing loss and abnormal behavior, such as head bobbing and an unbalanced gait [47, 48]. Although behavior is normal in heterozygous mice with the $Atp2b2$ mutant allele series, mice heterozygous for both $Atp2b2^{dfw\text{-}2J}$ and $Atp2b2^{dfw\text{-}i5}$ null alleles exhibit a significant increase in ABR threshold and progress from normal hearing to severe hearing loss at 5–10 weeks of age with $Cdh23^{ahl}$ allele homozygosity [8, 48, 49]. We recently found a similar situation in early-onset progressive hearing loss in mice heterozygous for the Jackson shaker $Ush1g^{js}$ mutation [50] of the $Ush1g/Sans$ gene, and we confirmed that the early-onset progressive hearing loss is strongly linked with homozygosity of the $Cdh23^{ahl}$ allele through genetic analysis (data not shown). Additionally, modification of the hearing phenotype due to $Cdh23^{ahl}$ allele homozygosity has been reported in several knockout (KO) mice of genes associated with hearing. Although conditional KO $Actb^{flox/flox}$ mice of the actin-β gene $Actb$ had shortened stereocilia, the phenotype depends on homozygosity of the $Cdh23^{ahl}$ allele [34]. Moreover, Johnson et al. [51] reported that AHL and hair cell loss are accelerated in KO mice by the antioxidant enzyme superoxide dismutase 1 soluble $Sod1$ by homozygosity of the $Cdh23^{ahl}$ allele. Thus, the CDH23 allele functions to maintain hearing as a susceptible modifier.

AHL-Resistance Effect of the *ahl3* Locus in $Cdh23^{ahl}$ Homozygosity Defined by Phenotypic Analysis of the C57BL/6J-Chr 17$^{MSM/Ms}$ Consomic Strain

Although homozygosity of the $Cdh23^{ahl}$ allele is a strong susceptibility modifier in mice, as mentioned above, we previously found that the intersubspecific C57BL/6J-Chr 17$^{MSM/Ms}$ consomic strain (fig. 3a) is resistant to AHL, despite having the $Cdh23^{ahl}$ mutation (fig. 3b) [52]. The C57BL/6J-Chr $^{\#MSM/Ms}$ consomic strain is an

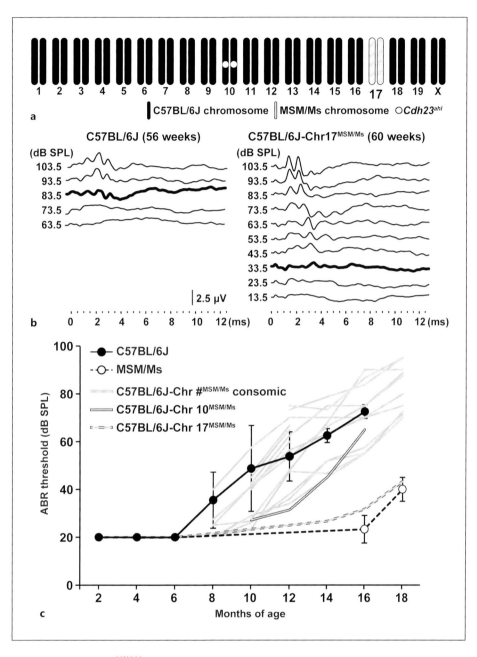

Fig. 3. C57BL/6J-Chr #[MSM/Ms] consomic strains modify the onset of AHL. **a** Chromosomal structure of a C57BL/6J-Chr 17[MSM/Ms] consomic mouse. **b** Representative ABR waveforms with a 10-kHz stimulus recorded from C57BL/6J and C57BL/6J-Chr17[MSM/Ms] mice at 56 and 60 weeks of age, respectively. The waveforms represent the ABR in response to tone-pip stimuli decreasing in intensity from 103.5 to 13.5 dB SPL. Bold lines represent the detected thresholds. **c** Variations in AHL onset among the C57BL/6J-Chr #[MSM/Ms] consomic strains. Data for the ABR thresholds of consomic strains are cited from our previous study [52].

inbred strain with one of its chromosomes replaced by the homologous chromosome from wild mouse *Mus musculus molossinus*-derived MSM/Ms in the C57BL/6J genetic background, which derives most of its genome from *M. m. domesticus* and enables the identification of QTLs on a particular chromosome because the appropriate consomic can be backcrossed to the C57BL/6J strain and then intercrossed; thus, C57BL/6J-Chr #[MSM/Ms] congenic progeny with recombination events in the MSM/Ms chromosome can be identified [53]. Using this approach, we produced several C57BL/6J-Chr 17[MSM/Ms] lines and detected a novel resistance modifier, named the *ahl3* locus, within a 14-Mb region on chromosome 17 [52, 54]. Moreover, our study indicated that congenic mice carrying the MSM/Ms-derived *ahl3* locus did not exhibit a permanent threshold shift after exposure to noise pressure at a high level. This result suggests that the *ahl3* locus is also associated with resistance to noise-induced hearing loss (NIHL) [54].

MSM/Ms mice maintain stable hearing from 1 to 16 months of age [52]. This stability may be explicable by the *Cdh23*[ahl] mutation, because MSM/Ms mice do not have the *Cdh23*[ahl] mutation. As expected, in C57BL/6J-Chr 10[MSM/Ms] consomic mice, which have the replacement MSM/Ms-derived chromosome 10, including the wild-type *Cdh23* allele, the ABR thresholds were significantly lower than in C57BL/6J mice (fig. 3c). However, the consomic mice exhibit AHL after 12 months of age (fig. 3c), suggesting that C57BL/6J mice have other modifiers for hearing in their genetic background. Interestingly, not only C57BL/6J-Chr 17[MSM/Ms] mice but also other consomic strains differ significantly from the host C57BL/6J strain across hearing ability. We measured the ABR thresholds of several consomic strains and found susceptibility in 1 strain and resistance in the other 3 strains, in addition to the C57BL/6J-Chr 10[MSM/Ms] and -Chr 17[MSM/Ms] strains (fig. 3c) [52]. A similar situation was observed in strain sets of another consomic strain,

C57BL/6J-Chr #[PWD/Ph]/ForeJ [55], which carries a chromosome from the *musculus* wild mouse-derived strain PWD/Ph introgressed into the C57BL/6J background (Mouse Phenome Database at The Jackson Laboratory, http://phenome. jax.org/). There are large genetic divergences, with more than one hundred million SNPs, between inbred strains such as C57BL/6J and wild *musculus*-derived strains [6]. Therefore, phenotypic differences from the host strain may be caused by allele-specific expression and splicing variants of transcripts from genomic polymorphisms on the substituted chromosome, including *cis*-regulatory regions, such as promoters, enhancers and insulators, acting as susceptibility and resistance modifiers. Moreover, the modification of hearing loss is believed to be caused by the reproduction of regulatory compatibility and incompatibility between the substituted chromosome and other chromosomes, such as *trans*-effects of the *cis*-variants. Thus, intersubspecific consomic strains may be useful models for understanding the network systems of genes and proteins, including expression, regulation and interactions, for hearing.

Concluding Remarks and Future Perspectives

Although the effect of *Cdh23*[ahl] on AHL has not been confirmed in humans and is not strong because the effect has been considerably weakened by chromosome substitution [52], it is the most common AHL mutation and genetic modifier in most inbred mouse strains. Moreover, the classical forward genetics approaches, which used inbred mice carrying *Cdh23*[ahl], are powerful methods for identifying the genetic modifiers and epistasis associated with AHL.

In future investigations, identification will efficiently increase by combining phenotypic QTL analysis (or genome-wide association study, GWAS) with expression QTL (eQTL) analysis to identify *cis*- and *trans*-effects. We propose that for QTL and eQTL analyses, mouse strains established for QTL analysis should be used, such as RI and consomic strains derived from the susceptibility and resistance strains in hearing loss because these strains facilitate the positional identification of loci and analysis of epistasis among loci. In particular, the identification of modifiers among wild-derived variants from other subspecies, such as *M. m. musculus, castaneus* and *molossinus*, should lead to the detection of disease modifiers that have been shaped by selection and might therefore be compatible with detection and function [1]. Moreover, mouse bioresources developed for large-scale systematic genetic analyses of complex traits, such as the Hybrid Mouse Diversity Panel (HMDP) and Collaborative Cross strains, will become useful for identifying genetic modifiers in hearing loss. Although there are strengths and weaknesses in both strains for genetic analysis, they have advantages in terms of resolution, cost, coverage, and reproducibility in quantitative genetic analyses and GWAS of the millions of SNPs accumulated in the mouse inbred strains for functional genomics compared with using classical genetic crosses between the susceptible and resistant inbred strains [56]. Lavinsky et al. [57] demonstrated that NADPH oxidase-3 *Nox3* is a critical gene for susceptibility to noise-induced hearing loss by GWAS and eQTL analyses in the HMDP and previously demonstrated the power for identifying genes associated with NIHL. In addition, outbred populations, which descend from several classical inbred strains, such as heterogeneous stocks, diversity outbred stocks and the UM-HET4 strain, will also become useful models for genetic analyses and the identification of genetic modifiers considering the heterogeneity of the human population [56, 58]. Indeed, Schacht et al. [58] identified several loci associated with AHL and NIHL by QTL mapping using UM-HET4 mice, which were established by 4-way crosses involving 4 inbred strains, 129S1/SvImJ, C3H/HeJ, FVB/NJ, and MOLF/EiJ.

In addition, the mouse models are useful for in vivo confirmation of genetic modifiers of hearing loss using reverse genetics approaches. Complementation experiments mediated by BAC transgenesis can confirm whether a candidate mutation identified by a forward genetics approach is responsible for modifying hearing loss [e.g. 33, 50]. Although archives generated by mouse N-ethyl-N-nitrosourea (ENU) mutagenesis can be used for gene-driven screening of mutant mice with genetic modifiers identified by forward genetics approaches in humans and mice, we believe that the recently developed genome editing CRISPR/Cas system will become useful for confirming candidate genes and mutations and functional analyses of genetic modifiers because this system can conveniently manipulate mutations to more accurately mimicking specific features of human hearing loss [59]. For example, biological functions can be analyzed by the phenotypic analysis of mice modified with polymorphisms identified in GWAS in humans. Moreover, the genome-editing system will enable further genetic analysis of phenotypic modifiers because a given mutation can be transferred into different genetic backgrounds without the restrictions of inbred mouse strains.

Acknowledgements

We thank Hiromichi Yonekawa for critical review of this manuscript. We also thank Rie Hayashi and Shinya Ishizaka, Leica Microsystems K.K., for helping with STED imaging (fig. 1c). This work was financially supported by JSPS KAKENHI (Grants-in-Aid for Scientific Research B, Grant Numbers 23300160 and 15H04291, Y.K.; Grant-in-Aid for JSPS Fellows, Grant Number 14J06119, Y.M.).

References

1 Hamilton BA, Yu BD: Modifier genes and the plasticity of genetic networks in mice. PLoS Genet 2012;8:e1002644.

2 Fransen E, Lemkens N, Van Laer L, Van Camp G: Age-related hearing impairment (ARHI): environmental risk factors and genetic prospects. Exp Gerontol 2003;38:353–359.

3 Johnson KR, Zheng QY, Noben-Trauth K: Strain background effects and genetic modifiers of hearing in mice. Brain Res 2006;1091:79–88.

4 Kikkawa Y, Seki Y, Okumura K, Ohshiba Y, Miyasaka Y, et al: Advantages of a mouse model for human hearing impairment. Exp Anim 2012;61:85–98.

5 Keane TM, Goodstadt L, Danecek P, White MA, Wong K, et al: Mouse genomic variation and its effect on phenotypes and gene regulation. Nature 2011; 477:289–294.

6 Takada T, Ebata T, Noguchi H, Keane TM, Adams DJ, et al: The ancestor of extant Japanese fancy mice contributed to the mosaic genomes of classical inbred strains. Genome Res 2013;23: 1329–1338.

7 Zheng QY, Johnson KR, Erway LC: Assessment of hearing in 80 inbred strains of mice by ABR threshold analyses. Hear Res 1999;130:94–107.

8 Noben-Trauth K, Zheng QY, Johnson KR: Association of cadherin 23 with polygenic inheritance and genetic modification of sensorineural hearing loss. Nat Genet 2003;35:21–23.

9 Di Palma F, Holme RH, Bryda EC, Belyantseva IA, Pellegrino R, et al: Mutations in Cdh23, encoding a new type of cadherin, cause stereocilia disorganization in waltzer, the mouse model for Usher syndrome type 1D. Nat Genet 2001;27:103–107.

10 Bolz H, von Brederlow B, Ramírez A, Bryda EC, Kutsche K, et al: Mutation of CDH23, encoding a new member of the cadherin gene family, causes Usher syndrome type 1D. Nat Genet 2001;27:108–112.

11 Pan L, Zhang M: Structures of Usher syndrome 1 proteins and their complexes. Physiology 2012;27:25–42.

12 Siemens J, Lillo C, Dumont RA, Reynolds A, Williams DS, et al: Cadherin 23 is a component of the tip link in hair-cell stereocilia. Nature 2004;428:950–955.

13 Gillespie PG, Müller U: Mechanotransduction by hair cells: models, molecules, and mechanisms. Cell 2009;139:33–44.

14 Kazmierczak P, Sakaguchi H, Tokita J, Wilson-Kubalek EM, Milligan RA, et al: Cadherin 23 and protocadherin 15 interact to form tip-link filaments in sensory hair cells. Nature 2007;449:87–91.

15 Sotomayor M, Weihofen WA, Gaudet R, Corey DP: Structure of a force-conveying cadherin bond essential for inner-ear mechanotransduction. Nature 2012; 492:128–132.

16 Ahmed ZM, Riazuddin S, Bernstein SL, Ahmed Z, Khan S, et al: Mutations of the protocadherin gene PCDH15 cause Usher syndrome type 1F. Am J Hum Genet 2001;69:25–34.

17 Alagramam KN, Murcia CL, Kwon HY, Pawlowski KS, Wright CG, Woychik RP: The mouse Ames waltzer hearing-loss mutant is caused by mutation of Pcdh15, a novel protocadherin gene. Nat Genet 2001;27:99–102.

18 Lagziel A, Ahmed ZM, Schultz JM, Morell RJ, Belyantseva IA, Friedman TB: Spatiotemporal pattern and isoforms of cadherin 23 in wild type and waltzer mice during inner ear hair cell development. Dev Biol 2005;280:295–306.

19 Michel V, Goodyear RJ, Weil D, Marcotti W, Perfettini I, et al: Cadherin 23 is a component of the transient lateral links in the developing hair bundles of cochlear sensory cells. Dev Biol 2005;280:281–294.

20 Johnson KR, Erway LC, Cook SA, Willott JF, Zheng QY: A major gene affecting age-related hearing loss in C57BL/6J mice. Hear Res 1997;114:83–92.

21 Kane KL, Longo-Guess CM, Gagnon LH, Ding D, Salvi RJ, Johnson KR: Genetic background effects on age-related hearing loss associated with Cdh23 variants in mice. Hear Res 2012;283:80–88.

22 Keithley EM, Canto C, Zheng QY, Fischel-Ghodsian N, Johnson KR: Age-related hearing loss and the ahl locus in mice. Hear Res 2004;188:21–28.

23 Miyasaka Y, Suzuki S, Ohshiba Y, Watanabe K, Sagara Y, et al: Compound heterozygosity of the functionally null Cdh23v-ngt and hypomorphic Cdh23ahl alleles leads to early-onset progressive hearing loss in mice. Exp Anim 2013;62: 333–346.

24 Nagtegaal AP, Spijker S, Crins TT, Neuro-Bsik Mouse Phenomics Consortium, Borst JG: A novel QTL underlying early-onset, low-frequency hearing loss in BXD recombinant inbred strains. Genes Brain Behav 2012;11:911–920.

25 Schwander M, Xiong W, Tokita J, Lelli A, Elledge HM, et al: A mouse model for nonsyndromic deafness (DFNB12) links hearing loss to defects in tip links of mechanosensory hair cells. Proc Natl Acad Sci U S A 2009;106:5252–5257.

26 Someya S, Xu J, Kondo K, Ding D, Salvi RJ, et al: Age-related hearing loss in C57BL/6J mice is mediated by Bak-dependent mitochondrial apoptosis. Proc Natl Acad Sci U S A 2009;106:19432–19437.

27 Someya S, Yu W, Hallows WC, Xu J, Vann JM, et al: Sirt3 mediates reduction of oxidative damage and prevention of age-related hearing loss under caloric restriction. Cell 2010;143:802–812.

28 Zheng QY, Ding D, Yu H, Salvi RJ, Johnson KR: A locus on distal chromosome 10 ahl4 affecting age-related hearing loss in A/J mice. Neurobiol Aging 2009; 30:1693–1705.

29 Johnson KR, Zheng QY, Weston MD, Ptacek LJ, Noben-Trauth K: The Mass1frings mutation underlies early onset hearing impairment in BUB/BnJ mice, a model for the auditory pathology of Usher syndrome IIC. Genomics 2005;85:582–590.

30 Johnson KR, Longo-Guess C, Gagnon LH, Yu H, Zheng QY: A locus on distal chromosome 11 ahl8 and its interaction with Cdh23ahl underlie the early onset, age-related hearing loss of DBA/2J mice. Genomics 2008;92:219–225.

31 Johnson KR, Zheng QY: Ahl2, a second locus affecting age-related hearing loss in mice. Genomics 2002;80:461–464.

32 Suzuki S, Ishikawa M, Ueda T, Ohshiba Y, Miyasaka Y, et al: Quantitative trait loci on chromosome 5 for susceptibility to frequency-specific effects on hearing in DBA/2J mice. Exp Anim 2015;64: 241–251.

33 Shin JB, Longo-Guess CM, Gagnon LH, Saylor KW, Dumont RA, et al: The R109H variant of fascin-2, a developmentally regulated actin crosslinker in hair-cell stereocilia, underlies early-onset hearing loss of DBA/2J mice. J Neurosci 2010;30:9683–9694.

34 Perrin BJ, Strandjord DM, Narayanan P, Henderson DM, Johnson KR, Ervasti JM: β-Actin and fascin-2 cooperate to maintain stereocilia length. J Neurosci 2013;33:8114–8121.

35 Skradski SL, Clark AM, Jiang H, White HS, Fu YH, Ptácek LJ: A novel gene causing a Mendelian audiogenic mouse epilepsy. Neuron 2001;31:537–544.

36 Weston MD, Luijendijks MWJ, Humphreys KD, Mollers C, Kimberling WJ: Mutations in the *VLGR1* gene implicate G-protein signaling in the pathogenesis of Usher syndrome type II. Am J Hum Genet 2004;74:357–366.

37 McGee J, Goodyear RJ, McMillan DR, Stauffer EA, Holt JR, et al: The very large G-protein-coupled receptor VLGR1: a component of the ankle link complex required for the normal development of auditory hair bundles. J Neurosci 2006; 26:6543–6553.

38 Michalski N, Michel V, Bahloul A, Lefèvre G, Barral J, et al: Molecular characterization of the ankle-link complex in cochlear hair cells and its role in the hair bundle functioning. J Neurosci 2007;27: 6478–6488.

39 Zallocchi M, Delimont D, Meehan DT, Cosgrove D: Regulated vesicular trafficking of specific PCDH15 and VLGR1 variants in auditory hair cells. J Neurosci 2012;32:13841–13859.

40 Zallocchi M, Meehan DT, Delimont D, Rutledge J, Gratton MA, et al: Role for a novel Usher protein complex in hair cell synaptic maturation. PLoS One 2012; 7:e30573.

41 Han X, Ge R, Xie G, Li P, Zhao X, et al: Caspase-mediated apoptosis in the cochleae contributes to the early onset of hearing loss in A/J mice. ASN Neuro 2015;7:1759091415573985.

42 Johnson KR, Zheng QY, Bykhovskaya Y, Spirina O, Fischel-Ghodsian N: A nuclear-mitochondrial DNA interaction affecting hearing impairment in mice. Nat Genet 2001;27:191–194.

43 Johnson KR, Gagnon LH, Longo-Guess C, Kane KL: Association of a citrate synthase missense mutation with age-related hearing loss in A/J mice. Neurobiol Aging 2012;33:1720–1729.

44 Cheng TL, Liao CC, Tsai WH, Lin CC, Yeh CW, et al: Identification and characterization of the mitochondrial targeting sequence and mechanism in human citrate synthase. J Cell Biochem 2009; 107:1002–1015.

45 Kokotas H, Petersen MB, Willems PJ: Mitochondrial deafness. Clin Genet 2007;71:379–391.

46 Han C, Someya S: Mouse models of age-related mitochondrial neurosensory hearing loss. Mol Cell Neurosci 2013;55: 95–100.

47 Street VA, McKee-Johnson JW, Fonseca RC, Tempel BL, Noben-Trauth K: Mutations in a plasma membrane Ca^{2+}-ATPase gene cause deafness in deafwaddler mice. Nat Genet 1998;19:390–394.

48 Noben-Trauth K, Zheng QY, Johnson KR, Nishina PM: *mdfw*: a deafness susceptibility locus that interacts with deaf waddler *dfw*. Genomics 1997;44:266–272.

49 Watson CJ, Tempel BL: A new *Atp2b2* deafwaddler allele, *dfw* (i5), interacts strongly with *Cdh23* and other auditory modifiers. Hear Res 2013;304:41–48.

50 Kikkawa Y, Shitara H, Wakana S, Kohara Y, Takada T, et al: Mutations in a new scaffold protein *Sans* cause deafness in Jackson shaker mice. Hum Mol Genet 2013;12:453–461.

51 Johnson KR, Yu H, Ding D, Jiang H, Gagnon LH, Salvi RJ: Separate and combined effects of *Sod1* and *Cdh23* mutations on age-related hearing loss and cochlear pathology in C57BL/6J mice. Hear Res 2010;268:85–92.

52 Nemoto M, Morita Y, Mishima Y, Takahashi S: Nomura T, et al: *Ahl3*, a third locus on mouse chromosome 17 affecting age-related hearing loss. Biochem Biophys Res Commun 2004;324:1283–1288.

53 Takada T, Mita A, Maeno A, Sakai T, Shitara H, et al: Mouse inter-subspecific consomic strains for genetic dissection of quantitative complex traits. Genome Res 2008;18:500–508.

54 Morita Y, Hirokawa S, Kikkawa Y, Nomura T, Yonekawa H, et al: Fine mapping of *Ahl3* affecting both age-related and noise-induced hearing loss. Biochem Biophys Res Commun 2007;355: 117–121.

55 Gregorová S, Divina P, Storchova R, Trachtulec Z, Fotopulosova V, et al: Mouse consomic strains: exploiting genetic divergence between *Mus m. musculus* and *Mus m. domesticus* subspecies. Genome Res 2008;18:509–515.

56 Flint J, Eskin E: Genome-wide association studies in mice. Nat Rev Genet 2012;13:807–817.

57 Lavinsky J, Crow AL, Pan C, Wang J, Aaron KA, et al: Genome-wide association study identifies *Nox3* as a critical gene for susceptibility to noise-induced hearing loss. PLoS Genet 2015;11: e1005094.

58 Schacht J, Altschuler R, Burke DT, Chen S, Dolan D, et al: Alleles that modulate late life hearing in genetically heterogeneous mice. Neurobiol Aging 2012;33: 1842.e15–e29.

59 Platt RJ, Chen S, Zhou Y, Yim MJ, Swiech L, et al: CRISPR-Cas9 knockin mice for genome editing and cancer modeling. Cell 2014;159:440–455.

60 Latoche JR, Neely HR, Noben-Trauth K: Polygenic inheritance of sensorineural hearing loss *Snhl2*, *-3*, and *-4* and organ of Corti patterning defect in the ALR/LtJ mouse strain. Hear Res 2011;275:150–159.

Yoshiaki Kikkawa, PhD
Mammalian Genetics Project, Department of Genome Medicine
Tokyo Metropolitan Institute of Medical Science
2-1-6 Kamikitazawa, Setagaya-ku, Tokyo 156-8506 (Japan)
E-Mail kikkawa-ys@igakuken.or.jp

Vona B, Haaf T (eds): Genetics of Deafness. Monogr Hum Genet. Basel, Karger, 2016, vol 20, pp 110–131
(DOI: 10.1159/000444569)

Using Zebrafish to Study Human Deafness and Hearing Regeneration

Gaurav K. Varshney[1] · Wuhong Pei[1] · Shawn M. Burgess

Translational and Functional Genomics Branch, National Human Genome Research Institute, National Institutes of Health, Bethesda, Md., USA

Abstract

Since the publication of the first draft of the human genome sequence in 2001, there has been an explosion in the number of genes associated with human genetic diseases, including those involved in human deafness. Clinical studies, genome-wide association studies, and exome resequencing have all added to the ever-expanding candidate list of genes with a role in hearing. Because human genetic data is primarily correlative, this explosion of data has increased the need for more efficient approaches to confirm these candidate genes in a model system. In addition, as our understanding of stem cells and genome editing advances, the potential for restoring hearing through regenerative medicine increases. This review highlights the role zebrafish can play as a model for human deafness, and also its potential role in discovering regenerative medicine therapies to restore lost hearing. © 2016 S. Karger AG, Basel

Hearing loss is one of the most common quality-of-life pathologies affecting the human population. Approximately 2–3 of every 1,000 newborns have a detectable level of hearing loss in one or both ears, and more than 10% of the American population over 18 years of age are suffering with some level of hearing loss, with a clear progression in hearing loss as the person ages (National Institute on Deafness and Other Communication Disorders, http://www.nidcd.nih.gov/health/statistics/Pages/quick.aspx). At age 70 and above, over 50% of the population has measurable hearing loss.

Hearing is mediated by a sensory epithelium containing acoustic mechanosensory receptors called hair cells and a second cell type known as supporting cells located in the cochlea of the inner ear [1]. This epithelium converts sound waves into electrical impulses ultimately interpreted as hearing in the brain. Hearing loss can be caused by many factors such as exposure to loud noise (https://www.nidcd.nih.gov/staticresources/health/hearing/NIDCD-Noise-Induced-Hearing-Loss.pdf), ototoxic chemicals (aminoglycoside antibiotics, cisplatin) [2], infection [3], or head injury [4, 5]. Genetic factors are likely to play an important role in disease pathogenesis, and recent work has attempted to identify genes that make individuals more susceptible to progressive hearing loss [6].

Like most fish, zebrafish have two related sensory organs that utilize the mechanosensory hair cell receptors: (1) the inner ear similar to mammalian ears used to detect sound, gravity, and motion, and (2) the lateral line [7], a fish- and am-

[1] G.K.V. and W.P. contributed equally to this work.

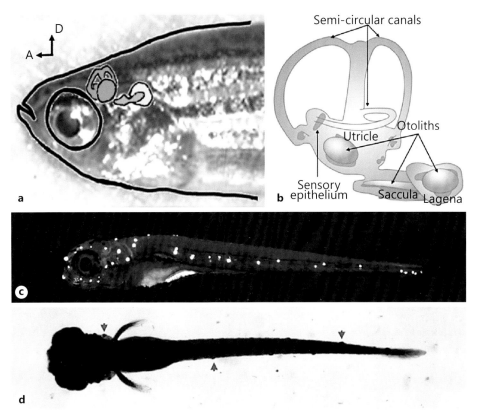

Fig. 1. The inner ear and the lateral line in zebrafish. **a** A bright field image of an adult zebrafish head, with inner ear structure illustrated. The adult fish is oriented in a lateral view, with the nose on the left. The utricle and semicircular canals are highlighted in green, the saccula in blue, and the lagena in yellow. **b** A cartoon illustration of the structure of the adult zebrafish inner ear. The utricle is involved in vestibular functions, the saccula is primarily hearing, and the lagena is an indeterminate mixture of hearing and vestibular functions. **c** A fluorescent image of a zebrafish larva, with hair cells stained using the fluorescent dye Yopro-1. The larva is oriented in a lateral view, with head on the left. Each white dot along the body and head is a cluster of hair cells centered in a neuromast. **d** A bright field image of a zebrafish larva. The larva is oriented in a ventral view, with head on the left. Arrows point to examples of the hair cell-containing neuromasts localized superficially on the skin (visible as small bumps). A = Anterior; D = dorsal.

phibian-specific organ used to detect water flow over the surface of the body (fig. 1). The neuromast consists of clusters of hair cells and supporting cells along the side of the body with each cell type having similar molecular signature to the matching cells in the mammalian inner ear.

Intense sound or toxic chemical exposure can damage or kill hair cells which are often more sensitive to injury than the surrounding epithelium [8, 9]. In mammals, these sensory hair cells can only repair themselves if the damage is modest; however, if the damage is significant, apoptosis is triggered in the hair cells. Only non-mammalian vertebrates such as fish or frogs can fully regenerate damaged hearing. In mammals, such as humans, the damage is permanent. Typically, in fish, the supporting cells re-enter mitosis and hair cells differentiate from these activated supporting cells, rapidly and completely restoring full hearing [7]. In recent years, zebrafish has been increasingly used as a model for human disease, including human deafness, because its genome has been fully sequenced [10], and targeted gene inactivation has become commonplace [11]. Zebrafish are also advantageous in terms of visualizing defects in the inner ear as their eggs are fertilized externally and the larvae are optically transparent for the first several days of development, allowing direct observation of the sensory epithelium of the inner ear. In mouse, sensory hair cells are not as directly accessible for either observation or manipulation, and dissection of the inner ear is technically challenging. Because of this general utility, zebrafish is being increasingly used as a model system for human deafness and for studying the factors involved in hearing regeneration. There are many reviews outlining the development of hair cells in zebrafish [12–16]; therefore, in this review, we will focus on recent advances in the use of zebrafish to directly model known human deafness genes and recent advances in our understanding of hearing regeneration in non-mammalian vertebrates.

Zebrafish as a Model for Human Deafness

In nonsyndromic deafness, hearing loss is not accompanied by other symptoms. Approximately 2 of 3 genetic hearing loss conditions are nonsyndromic in nature. According to the Hereditary Hearing loss website (http://hereditaryhearingloss. org), there are more than 100 genes associated with nonsyndromic hearing loss. Of the nonsyndromic deafness cases, 70% are classified as autosomal recessive deafness (DFNB) and 20% as autosomal dominant deafness (DFNA). The remaining cases are caused by X-linked or mitochondrial genetic mutations. In syndromic deafness, the hearing loss is usually associated with other clinical manifestations such as blindness or dysmorphic craniofacial features. The syndromic forms of deafness account for one-third of all hearing loss cases.

In most cases, the genetic evidence for deafness in humans is very good; however, functional validation for most of the candidate genes has not been done. The most common method of validat-

ing candidate gene function is to generate a gene knockout in the homologous gene in a model organism; for example, 70% of human genes have orthologs in zebrafish [10]. We have summarized all genes in zebrafish that have an orthologous human gene related to nonsyndromic deafness in table 1. Several large-scale mutagenesis screens have identified multiple genes essential for balance and hearing in zebrafish [17–20]. The screens mainly identified genes based on morphology such as otic placode specification, otolith formation, size and shape of otic vesicle, etc. Approximately 40 such genes were identified for inner ear development [18, 21]. A second approach was based on screening locomotion and behavior of larvae that had normal otic vesicle morphology. This approach identified 17 mutants representing 9 genes where mutations caused the 'circler' phenotype. These mutants swam in an erratic fashion when provided with tactile stimulation and did not display an escaping startle response when provided with an acoustic tapping sound. This group of mutants was called the circler mutants [19]. Eight of the circler mutants (*sputnik, mariner, orbiter, mercury, gemini, skylab, astronaut,* and *cosmonaut)* were further investigated for vestibular function defects, acoustic startle reflex and microphonics [17]. Although many mutations affecting hair cell development have been identified, only a fraction of these are linked to disease pathology. However, the circler class of mutants have a strong correlation with deafness-associated genes and has proven to be a more effective method for identifying models of human deafness than the gross morphological approaches. The following sections will describe the known human deafness genes that have a published zebrafish disease model.

Myosin VIIA (MYO7A)

In humans, *MYO7A* has been implicated in both syndromic and nonsyndromic deafness. Liu et al. [22] identified a heterozygous mutation in the

Table 1. Zebrafish orthologs of known nonsyndromic deafness genes

Human deafness locus	Human gene	Zebrafish gene(s)	Zebrafish model	References
DFNA20/26	ACTG1	–	–	[107, 108]
DFNB44	ADCY1	adcy1a, adcy1b	yes	[47]
DFNB93	CABP2	cabp2a, cabp2b	–	[109]
DFNA44	CCDC50	–	–	[110]
DFNB12	CDH23	cadherin-like 23	yes	[32, 111]
DFNB48	CIB2	cib2	–	[112]
DFNB29	CLDN14	–	–	[113]
DFNB102	CLIC5	clic5a, clic5b	–	[114]
DFNA9	COCH	coch	–	[115, 116]
DFNB53, DFNA13	COL11A2	col11a2	–	[117]
DFNA40	CRYM	crym	–	[118]
DFNA5	DFNA5	dfna5a, dfna5b	yes	[11, 37, 38]
DFNA1	DIAPH1	–	–	[119]
DFNB88	ELMOD3	elmod3	–	[120]
DFNB102	EPS8	eps8l3, eps8l1	–	[121]
DFNB36	ESPN	espn, espnl	–	[122]
DFNB35	ESRRB	esrrb	–	[123]
DFNA10	EYA4	eya4	–	[124]
DFNB15/72/95	GIPC3	gipc3	–	[125–127]
DFNB1A, DFNA3A	GJB2	–	–	[128–130]
DFNB91, DFNA2B	GJB3	cx35.4	–	[131]
DFNB1B, DFNA3B	GJB6	cx30.3	–	[132]
DFNB82	GPSM2	gpsm2	–	[133]
DFNA28	GRHL2	grhl2a, grhl2b	yes	[39–41]
DFNB25	GRXCR1	grxcr1	–	[134]
DFNB101	GRXCR2	grxcr2	–	[135]
DFNB39	HGF	hgfa, hgfb	–	[136]
DFNB42	ILDR1	ildr1a, ildr1b	–	[49]
DFNB89	KARS	kars	–	[137]
DFNA2A	KCNQ4	kcnq4	–	[138]
DFNB66/67	LHFPL5	lhfpl5a, lhfpl5b	–	[139–141]
DFNB77	LOXHD1	loxhd1a, loxhd1b	–	[142]
DFNB63	LRTOMT/COMT2	lrtomt	–	
DFNB49	MARVELD2	marveld2a, marveld2b	–	[143]
DFNA50	MIRN96	mir96	yes	[144]
DFNB74	MSRB3	msrb3	yes	[1, 145, 146]
DFNA4	MYH14, CEACAM16	myh14	–	[147]
DFNA17	MYH9	myh9a, myh9b	–	[148]
DFNB3	MYO15A	myo15aa, myo15ab	–	[149]
DFNB30	MYO3A	myo3a	–	[150]
DFNB37, DFNA22	MYO6	myo6a, myo6b	yes	[29–31, 151]
DFNB2, DFNA11	MYO7A, MYO7A	myo7aa, myo7ab	yes	[152, 153]
DFNB22	OTOA	si:dkey-71b5.7	–	[154]
DFNB9	OTOF, OTOG	otofa, otofb, otog	yes	[155–158]
DFNB84	OTOGL	otogl	–	[158]
DFNA41	P2RX2	p2rx2	–	[159]
DFNB23	PCDH15	pcdh15a, pcdh15b	yes	[28, 37]
DFNB59	PJVK	dfnb59	–	[160]
DFNB70	PNPT1	pnpt1	–	[161]

Table 1. Continued

Human deafness locus	Human gene	Zebrafish gene(s)	Zebrafish model	References
DFNX2 (DFN3)	POU3F4	–	–	[162]
DFNA15	POU4F3	pou4f3	–	[163]
DFNX1 (DFN2)	PRPS1	prps1a, prps1b	–	[164]
DFNB84	PTPRQ	ptprq	–	[165]
DFNB24	RDX, SERPINB6	msna, msnb	–	[166, 167]
DFNA23	SIX1	six1a, six1b	–	[168]
DFNA25	SLC17A8	slc17a8/vglut3	–	[169, 170]
DFNB4	SLC26A4	slc26a4	–	[171]
DFNB61	SLC26A5	slc26a5	–	[172]
DFNA64	SMAC/DIABLO	diabloa	–	[173]
DFNX4 (DFN6)	SMPX	smpx	–	[174, 175]
DFNB16	STRC	–	–	[176]
DFNB76	SYNE4	–	–	[177]
DFNB86, DFNA65	TBC1D24	tbc1d24	–	[178]
DFNB21, DFNA8/12	TECTA	tecta	–	[179, 180]
DFNA51	TJP2	tjp2a, tjp2b	–	[181]
DFNB7/11, DFNA36	TMC1	tmc1	–	[182]
DFNB6	TMIE	tmie	yes	[43, 46]
DFNB8/10	TMPRSS3	tmprss3a, tmprss3b	–	[183]
DFNA56	TNC	tnc	–	[184]
DFNB79	TPRN	tprn	–	[185, 186]
DFNB28	TRIOBP	triobpa, tiobpb	–	[187, 188]
DFNB98	TSPEAR	tspear	–	[189]
DFNB18	USH1C	ush1c	–	[190, 191]
DFNA6/14/38	WFS1	wfs1a, wfs1b	–	[192, 193]
DFNB31	WHRN	dfnb31a, dfn31b	–	[194]

MYO7A gene in a Japanese family with nonsyndromic DFNA11, and later a different heterozygous mutation was also found in a Dutch family [23]. Mutations in *MYO7A* were also detected in families with nonsyndromic DFNB2 [22, 24, 25]. In addition, mutations in *MYO7A* have been identified in patients with Usher syndrome type 1B [24, 26]. In zebrafish, one of the circler mutants, *mariner*, was shown to have mutations in the homologous zebrafish *myo7aa* gene [27]. *myo7aa* encodes an unconventional myosin and is expressed in the sensory hair cells of the inner ear and in the neuromasts of the lateral line system. Zebrafish *mariner* mutant embryos show defective hair cell bundles in the inner ear. These mutants do not have acoustic vibrational sensitivity and exhibit reduced or no hair cell potentials. The strongest allele of *myo7aa*

showed severe splaying of the hair cell bundles. Zebrafish m*yo7aa* phenotypes are similar in nature to the *shaker-1* mutants in mouse, which also show defective hair cell bundles [28]. These congruent data demonstrate the conservation of gene function across human, mouse and zebrafish. The mariner *(myo7aa)* mutant was the first example of modeling genetic human deafness in zebrafish and went a long way towards demonstrating the utility of using zebrafish to model human deafness.

Myosin VI *(MYO6)*

The *MYO6* gene encodes the myosin VI protein. As a general rule, myosins are involved in transporting molecules within cells and interact with filamentous actin. Myosins are believed to move along long filaments of actin transporting other molecules. In humans, mutations in *MYO6* can cause both nonsyndromic autosomal recessive DFNB37 [29] and autosomal dominant deafness, DFNA22 [30]. Because of a genome duplication in the teleost lineages, 20% of the genes, including *myo6*, are duplicated in the zebrafish genome. *myo6a* is ubiquitously expressed during early stages of development, and is expressed in the gut, kidney and brain at later stages, while *myo6b* is mainly expressed in the sensory epithelium of the inner ear and lateral line throughout the development [31]. Mutations in *myo6b* caused vestibular defects and lack of an acoustic startle reflex in zebrafish larvae [31]. *myo6b* mutants also exhibited altered hair-cell morphology with irregular and disorganized hair bundles [31]; a similar phenotype is also seen in a mouse knockout model [30].

Cadherin-23 *(CDH23)*

The *CDH23* gene encodes the cadherin-23 protein, a member of the cadherin family of proteins involved in cell attachment. More than 20 mutations in *CDH23* have been identified in individuals with nonsyndromic DFNB12 or in Usher syndrome type 1D. In families with nonsyndromic deafness, missense mutations are always reported, while families with Usher syndrome can have nonsense, splice-site, missense, or frameshift mutations in *CDH23*. In zebrafish, positional cloning of the circler mutant *sputnik* showed that the phenotypes were due to a mutation in the zebrafish homolog of cadherin-23, *cdh23* [32]. In the *sputnik* mutants, hair bundles are absent and mechanotransduction is compromised [17]. Hair bundles are detached from their respective kinocilia, and different alleles show variable degrees of 'splaying' of the hair bundles. These mutants do not respond to sound and display an abnormal swimming pattern. Zebrafish *cdh23* mRNA is expressed as early as 24 hours post fertilization (hpf) in the developing ear and at later

stages is limited to the neuroepithelium of the inner ear and lateral line neuromasts. Cdh23 protein is localized near the tip of hair bundles, and *cdh23* mutants lack the tip-link structure essential for normal sound detection [32]. In the mouse, CDH23 proteins are an essential part of the functioning tip-link structure and are assumed to perform the same role in zebrafish [33].

Protocadherin-Related 15 *(PCDH15)*

Mutations in the *PCDH15* gene have been discovered in many families with Usher syndrome type 1D, 1F and DFNB23 [34–36]. In zebrafish, one of the mutants identified in the Tübingen screen, *orbiter*, showed a vestibular defect and did not respond to startle stimuli. These mutants also lacked measurable hair cell extracellular microphonic potential [17]. The gene mutated in *orbiter* was identified as protocadherin-related 15 *(pcdh15)*. In zebrafish, *pcdh15* is duplicated as *pcdh15a* and *pcdh15b*. The hearing phenotype is specifically attributed to mutations in *pcdh15a,* while *pcdh15b* has phenotypes disrupting eye function [28]. *pcdh15a* is expressed in the eye and developing mechanosensory hair cells at 24 hpf. At later stages, *pcdh15a* becomes restricted to the hair cells of the inner ear and lateral line neuromasts. The *pcdh15a* mutants showed splaying of hair bundles in the semicircular canal. The splaying was less severe in weaker alleles suggesting a role for Pcdh15a in maintaining connections between filaments in the hair cell bundles. The number of hair cells in the neuromast was also reduced in *pcdh15a* mutants. This phenotype is consistent with the human phenotype, and the human PCDH15 protein was shown to be localized in hair bundles [36]. Evidence in mammals revealed that *PCDH15* [28] and *CDH23* work together to form the tip links (the key structure for opening the gated channel during signal detection) of the hair cell bundles [33]. The fact that zebrafish *cdh23* and *pcdh15a* mutants have similar phenotypes is consistent with these findings.

Deafness, Autosomal Dominant 5 (DFNA5)

Mutations in the *DFNA5* gene were first identified in an extended Dutch family with nonsyndromic autosomal dominant hearing loss [37], and later more mutations were identified in other families. These mutations caused a truncated version of the DFNA5 protein. In zebrafish, *dfna5* is duplicated and has 2 copies, *dfna5a* and *dfna5b*. *dfna5b* is expressed ubiquitously before 20 hpf, and at 48 hpf, it is expressed in the brain and ear, mostly in the projections of the developing semicircular canals [38]. By 55 hpf, expression is more restricted to the ear. Morpholino-mediated knockdown of *dfna5b* caused ear and jaw phenotypes. Morphant animals have unfused ear columns (the tissues that fuse to form the semicircular canals) resulting in malformed semicircular canals. Higher doses of *dfna5b* morpholino also show abnormal jaw development, but that phenotype is not supported by the genetic mutation [11]. The molecular function of Dfna5b is not known, but it has been suggested that it could play an important role in the hyaluronic acid biosynthesis pathway and could act at the transcriptional level [38].

Grainyhead-Like 2 (GRHL2)

A mutation in *GRHL2* was found in a large American family with nonsyndromic DFNA28 [39] and was further confirmed in another large family [40]. *GRHL2* is a member of the grainyhead-like transcription factor family. In zebrafish, there are 3 members in this family, *grhl1*, *grhl2* and *grhl3*; *grhl2* has 2 copies, *grhl2a* and *grhl2b*. *grhl2b* expression was detected in the anterior lateral line primordium, the lateral line neuromasts and the otic vesicle [41]. *grhl2b* homozygous mutants showed defective hearing and an abnormal swimming pattern [41]. The mutant animals had a generally normal appearance

but had enlarged otocysts, thinner otic epithelium and either smaller or no otoliths. Overexpression of human or mouse *Grhl2* mRNA rescued the otolith defects, but the mutant forms of human *GRHL2* mRNA failed to rescue the phenotype. These results suggest that the role of *grhl2* in inner ear development is conserved in vertebrates, and the fact that the identified *GRHL2* mutation in DFNA28 patients does not rescue the zebrafish knockout, shows that the human variants are loss-of-function mutations [41]. This approach is becoming more frequently used as a method for demonstrating that human variants are nonfunctional. Even in cases where the zebrafish phenotype does not match the human disease well, complementation can still be used to demonstrate that the variant disrupts normal in vivo function. Han et al. [41] further showed that morpholino-mediated knockdown of *grhl1* and *grhl3* did not yield inner ear phenotypes; however, a more recent report suggests that morpholino-mediated knockdown of *grhl1* does affect inner ear development [12]. *grhl1* is expressed in a very similar pattern to that of *grhl2* in the anterior lateral line primordium, lateral line neuromasts, otic vesicle, and posterior lateral line primordium. The knockdown of *grhl1* showed various abnormal otolith phenotypes such as abnormal size, number and location. The number of neuromasts in the lateral line was also reduced, and embryos were not startle responsive. Liu et al. [42] also demonstrated that knockdown of *grhl1* causes desmosome disintegration and hair cell death by regulating the expression of demoglein-1 in otic vesicles.

Transmembrane Inner Ear (TMIE)

TMIE encodes the transmembrane inner ear protein, and many homozygous or compound heterozygous mutations in the *TMIE* gene have been reported in families with nonsyndromic DFNB6 [43, 44]. In zebrafish, *tmie* is expressed in the brain and developing otic vesicles as early as 26 hpf, and expression was also detected at later stages in the otic vesicle [45]. The homozygous mutant zebrafish developed normally and did not show any morphological phenotype. The hair cells appeared normal in shape and orientation, and the hair cells in the lateral line neuromast were also normal. However, the hair cells in mutant animals failed to incorporate the fluorescent dye 4-Di-2-ASP, which normally traverses through functional mechanotransduction channels. The lack of staining indicates defects in normal functionality of the receptors. In addition, electrophysiological experiments demonstrated defects in hair cell potential in mutant animals, and further studies showed that hair cells in the mutants contain short, disorganized hair bundles. The stereocilia neither had tip links nor insertional plaques, both of which are key parts of the transduction apparatus [46].

Adenylate Cyclase 1 (ADCY1)

A homozygous mutation in the adenylate cyclase 1 (ADCY1) gene was identified in the members of a Pakistani family with DFNB44 [47]. Adenylate cyclase is involved in the catalysis of ATP to cyclic AMP, an important component in the mechanotransduction of hearing [48]. There are 2 copies of the adcy1 gene in zebrafish, adcy1a and adcy1b. Morpholino-mediated knockdown of both adcy1a and adcy1b showed curved bodies, smaller eyes and brains. However, more than 90% adcy1a morphants possessed a normal startle response, while only a few adcy1b morphants responded to acoustic stimuli [47]. FM-143 fluorescent dye staining (a simple test of hair cell functionality in live embryos) was not endocytosed into hair cells of adcy1b morphants, while adcy1a morphants incorporated the dye normally, demonstrating that it is the adcy1b gene that is essential for hearing in zebrafish [47].

Immunoglobulin-Like Domain Containing Receptor 1 (ILDR1)

Two groups identified different homozygous mutations in the immunoglobulin-like domain containing receptor 1 (ILDR1) gene in members of 11 unrelated families with nonsyndromic DFNB42 [49]. Most of these mutations caused a protein truncation creating a loss-of-function allele. Zebrafish have 2 copies of ildr1, ildr1a and ildr1b. ildr1a has not been implicated in inner ear development, while ildr1b was expressed in the otic vesicle and the posterior lateral line primordium at 24 and 34 hpf, and from 48 to 96 hpf expression became more prominent in the inner ear and anterior lateral line neuromasts. Morpholino-mediated knockdown of ildr1b resulted in measurable hearing loss and an aberrant swimming pattern. Morphant embryos showed a delay in the development of the semicircular canals, a weak startle response and imbalanced swimming. The phenotype could be rescued by co-injecting mRNA encoding ildr1b. Morphant embryos also showed downregulation of the Na^+/K^+ ATPase encoding gene, atp1b2b. The ildr1b phenotype is partly rescued by ectopic expression of atp1b2b.

Family with Sequence Similarity 65, Member B (FAM65B)

Family with sequence similarity 65, member B (FAM65B) is a plasma membrane-associated protein of the hair cell stereocilia. Mutations in FAM65B were identified in 6 members of a Turkish family with profound sensorineural hearing loss [50]. The mutation found in these individuals caused an in-frame, exon 3-skipped variant. In zebrafish, fam65b mRNA was expressed in the otic vesicles of 72-hpf embryos. Morpholino-mediated knockdown of fam65b showed fewer hair cells in the inner ear as well as in the lateral line neuromasts. Acoustic measurements revealed that morphant embryos have a weaker microphonic response. The exact function of Fam65b is not yet known, but given its expression in the stereocilia of both outer and inner hair cells, it could be involved in the formation or differentiation of the mechanotransduction machinery [50].

Clarin-1 *(CLRN1)*

Mutations in Clarin-1 *(CLRN1)* are associated with Usher syndrome type IIIA. More than 10 mutations have been identified in this gene from different unrelated families with progressive vision and hearing loss [3, 4, 51]. Clarin-1 is a 4-pass membrane domain protein belonging to the tetraspanin family of proteins. In zebrafish, *clrn1* mRNA is expressed in mechanosensory hair cells and supporting cells of the inner ear as well as in the neuromasts of the lateral line [52]. Morpholino-mediated knockdown showed a reduced number of neuromasts in both the anterior and posterior lateral line. Morphant embryos did not take up FM-143 dye suggesting the hair cells do not have proper mechanotransduction activity. Biochemical evidence suggests that Clarin-1 interacts with Pcdh15a, an important component of tip links as described above. Mutations in the *PCDH15* gene are associated with nonsyndromic deafness and Usher syndrome type 1. Clrn1 was also shown to be involved in proper localization of synaptic components in hair cell synapses.

From both forward screening efforts and reverse genetic approaches (morpholinos), zebrafish has proven to have phenotypes consistent with the deafness seen in humans possessing mutations in the same genes. As genome editing approaches become more commonplace in zebrafish, it will be important to know just how often zebrafish mutations will confirm or recapitulate the deafness phenotypes seen in human patients. Having sufficient data between confirmed human disease alleles and the corresponding zebrafish knockout will allow better predictions on wheth-

er zebrafish mutant data can efficiently support new candidate deafness genes in the future [53–59].

Hearing Regeneration and Zebrafish

As most people are acutely aware either personally or from experience with aging family members, hearing loss in humans is generally progressive with age. Only 0.2–0.3% of infants are born with hearing deficiencies, but by the age of 75, over 50% of individuals will have measurable hearing loss (http://www.nidcd.nih.gov/health/statistics/Pages/quick.aspx). The primary reason for this progressive hearing loss is that humans and other mammals have no ability to regenerate hair cells after injury from environmental exposures (e.g. noise or ototoxic chemicals). In contrast, non-mammalian vertebrates have no such limitations; from fish [7, 14] to birds [60, 61], the majority of vertebrates can perfectly repair injuries to the sensory epithelium of the ear. In all cases, the new hair cells arise from the surrounding epithelium consisting of the supporting cells. The loss of hair cells triggers the supporting cells to either directly differentiate into hair cells, or to first enter into mitosis and then differentiate. The key difference between mammals and other vertebrates is the ability of these supporting cells to respond to hair cell injury. In mammals, there is no activation of the supporting cells after hair cell death, so receptor loss is permanent.

Therefore, the search for genes potentially capable of triggering hair cell regeneration must begin in vertebrate models that are capable of full hearing regeneration. As a result, zebrafish has been increasingly used to understand regeneration because it possesses several important properties that allow for sophisticated genetic approaches. First, it has a fully sequenced and annotated genome [10]; second, it now has efficient gene knockout techniques [11, 55–57]; and third, zebrafish possess a related organ known as the lat-

Fig. 2. A schematic representation of hair cell regeneration in zebrafish. **a** Hair cell regeneration through mitosis. **b** Hair cell regeneration through direct transdifferentiation. Hair cells are shown in blue. Support cells are shown in yellow. Nuclei are shown in brown. BM indicates the basement membrane. The stroma is shown by wavy lines. Moving from left to right in the pictures shows the steps in hair cell regeneration. On the left, the damaged hair cells are being extruded from the epithelium. The centers of the figures show that responding to hair cell damage support cells either go through mitosis (**a**) or direct transdifferentiation (**b**) in order to produce new hair cells. The right side shows newly regenerated hair cells acquire the cell identity and correctly reorganize the epithelium.

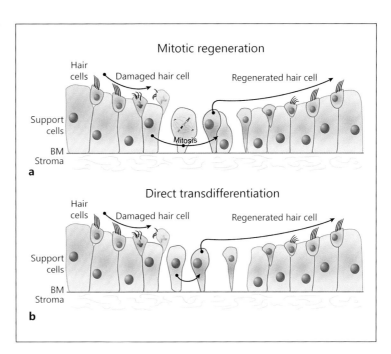

eral line (as do all fish), which has hair cells exposed to the aqueous environment. By targeting the hair cells of the lateral line with ototoxic chemicals, regeneration assays are simple and rapid.

Cellular Mechanisms

In zebrafish and many other vertebrates, regenerated hair cells arise from surrounding non-sensory supporting cells through 2 distinct mechanisms: proliferation or direct transdifferentiation [15, 62–66] (fig. 2). In zebrafish, these 2 mechanisms seem to be utilized under different injury conditions. In larval neuromasts, chemically-induced hair cell regeneration triggers supporting cell proliferation, as indicated by 3 lines of evidence. First, BrdU incorporation analysis revealed that hair cell ablation stimulates supporting cells to re-enter the cell cycle to produce new hair cells [63, 66, 67]. Second, gene expression analyses detected the activation of numerous genes associated with cell proliferation and cell cycle regulation in supporting cells [68, 69]. Third, chemical screening identified chemicals that promoted regeneration through increased supporting cell proliferation [70, 71]. It is also reported that in the zebrafish adult inner ear, noise-induced hair cell ablation also triggers the proliferation of supporting cells [72, 73]. However, in the developing larval zebrafish ear, laser ablation of hair cells induces regeneration involving direct transdifferentiation but no proliferation [74]. Furthermore, modest transdifferentiation was observed in the hair cell regeneration of zebrafish larvae exposed to a very low concentration of copper sulfate [75].

What triggers these 2 distinct mechanisms of hair cell regeneration requires further investigation. It could be associated with the identity of the ablated hair cells as determined by their location in the tissue, the release of injury signals may be different depending on how the cells were killed, the developmental stage, and/or the surrounding microenvironment. The ototoxin used for hair cell ablation could play a role, as different ototoxins have different efficiencies and modes of toxicity. Even the same ototoxin, when used at different concentrations, can have different effects on the survival and proliferation of surrounding cells [75]. In addition, the properties of the supporting cells matter. Since only a small fraction of supporting cells are used to replace the damaged hair cells, it raises questions about what makes that small fraction of supporting cells qualified for the task in non-mammalian vertebrates? Is it due to their relative position to the damaged hair cells, or their possession of specific signals that are able to instruct cell proliferation or transdifferentiation? Are these instruction signals from damaged hair cells or intrinsic to some supporting cells? Are supporting cells naturally heterogeneous, or is there a heterogeneous response caused by hair cell ablation? There is clearly still a great deal of work to be done in order to understand how these cells behave in their niche.

The importance of a third cell type in the lateral line known as mantle cells for hair cell regeneration remains unknown, largely because the mantle cell appears to be a cell type unique to the lateral line neuromast [13]. Gene expression analysis indicates there are genes triggered in the mantle cells during regeneration [69]. BrdU labeling analysis revealed many mantle cells became proliferative upon hair cell ablation, albeit at a lower frequency than that of the surrounding supporting cells [76]. Since a small population of mantle cells shared the same molecular identity as supporting cells [75], it suggests that mantle cells resume cell division upon hair cell ablation in order to compensate for the loss of supporting cells that will become hair cells. A well-known gene involved in stem cell maintenance and tissue regeneration, *stat3*, is strongly expressed in the mantle cells and is only later activated in all supporting cells after hair cell damage [77]. Such an expression pattern led us to suggest that the mantle cells represent the true stem cells in the lateral line [77]. Perhaps an analogous cell exists in the non-mam-

malian inner ear that behaves in the same, stem-cell like fashion. This model would place supporting cells in a state of 'pre-hair cell' potential, not specifically stem cells anymore but in a paused differentiation pathway that can be released by damage to nearby hair cells. Delta-Notch signaling is known to be involved in patterning the sensory epithelium, and the release of lateral inhibition of this signaling pathway is a potential mechanism for supporting cells to continue along the differentiation pathway to hair cells. While likely an oversimplification, there is a precedent for this model in skin homeostasis where stem cells divide, and some of those epidermal cells become committed to differentiate even as they continue to divide and amplify in number [78].

Epigenomics and/or Multi-Gene Effects

Just as single genetic mutations account for a fraction of common human diseases [20, 79], single causative genes have been found only for a small percentage of hearing disorders (http://www.nidcd.nih.gov/health/statistics/Pages/quick.aspx; http://hereditaryhearingloss.org). The majority of hearing loss is late onset and accumulated over time. An individual's susceptibility to hearing loss is almost certainly resulting from a combination of unknown genetic factors and environmental insults such as aging, noise or medication. Increasing evidence indicates that environmental insults not only result in mechanical or toxic damage to hair cells, but might cause changes in epigenetic programming [80–82]. Therefore, in addition to searching for genes associated with hearing regeneration, it will also be important to investigate relevant epigenetic changes.

Epigenetic research in zebrafish is at its early stage and there is not much progress to report in relation to hearing loss or regeneration. Some studies have shown that microRNA, DNA methylation and histone modification have an impact on hair cell development [83–86], but

Table 2. Hair cell regeneration-associated transcriptomics

Stage	Hair cell ablation	Tissue analyzed	Tissue purified by	Tissue used per sample	Transcript analysis	Genes associated with regeneration	Reference
Adult	sound	inner ear	dissection	inner ear tissue of 20 adult fish	microarray	1,721	[72]
Adult	sound	inner ear	dissection	inner ear tissue of 40 adult fish	digital gene expression	2,269	[77]
Larvae	neomycin	supporting and mantle cells	FACS	200 larvae	RNA-Seq	1,670	[68]
Larvae	CuSO$_4$	mantle cells	skin prep for FACS	skins of 50 larvae	microarray	8,569	[69]

there are no data on if the same processes are involved during regeneration. One of the advantages of zebrafish is that with a potential for hundreds of offspring, multi-gene phenomena can be more readily tested than in a mouse model. Similarly, epigenetic studies are becoming increasingly possible as organized efforts to systematically document epigenetic and transcribed elements in zebrafish (ZENCODE, http://www.birmingham.ac.uk/generic/zencode-itn/index.aspx) provide genome-wide information that can be applied to our understanding of complex interactions of genes and environment.

Assaying Hearing Regeneration in Zebrafish

Several studies have utilized zebrafish as a model to study genes expressed during hair cell regeneration, and each has identified a large set of differentially expressed genes [68, 69, 73, 77] (table 2). Various approaches to ablate hair cells and various ages of fish were used to analyze the transcripts. Despite the divergence in tissue preparation and in analysis methods, an overlapping set of genes has been discovered from these studies, including genes in the Notch, Wnt, Fgf, and Jak/Stat3 signaling pathways. These genes have also

been reported to be involved in the hair cell regeneration in other models [14] indicating shared mechanisms of hair cell regeneration across model systems. The major drawback with these studies is that the techniques used to purify the regenerating tissues are very invasive. The procedures involve microdissection, fluorescent-based cell sorting, or a combination of both. This likely induces a stress-damage response that alters or masks the expression of important regenerative genes. The solution to this limitation will rely on the development of new technologies that are capable of capturing transcripts more rapidly or are potentially able to sequence directly in situ using technologies such as FISSEQ [87].

Shared Mechanisms between Regeneration and Development

Several studies have shown that the process of hair cell regeneration utilizes similar signaling pathways to those used in initial hair cell development and differentiation. These signaling pathways include the Notch and Wnt pathways [15, 66, 68, 88–91]. In addition, several chemicals identified in drug screens performed on zebrafish embryos stimulated either hair cell regeneration or supernumerary hair cell development in the absence of injury, suggesting the same developmental pathways are being triggered in both cases [71]. This reactivation of developmental pathways was also observed during regeneration of other tissues in zebrafish [92], as well as in other model systems [90, 93]. These findings suggest that under certain conditions triggering specific differentiation pathways can result in some restoration of hair cell numbers.

Regeneration-Specific Genes

In contrast to the large number of genes that show differential expression during hearing regeneration, very few genes have been shown to be specifically necessary for hearing regeneration, i.e. genes that are only necessary for regeneration but do not have a role in normal development. One gene, *phoenix (pho)*, was identified that specifically impairs hair cell regeneration but is not involved in normal development or patterning [67]. *pho* is highly expressed in the supporting cells of the lateral line neuromasts, and *pho* mutants displayed a severe reduction of supporting cell proliferation during regeneration. Since *pho* is a novel gene with no obvious homologs, its molecular function remains unclear. The *stat3* pathway [77] and histone deacetylases (HDAC) [94] have been reported playing a role in hair cell regeneration. However, results were obtained from morpholino or pharmaceutical approaches, and given recent evidence that morpholino-generated phenotypes are often misleading [59], these results will need to be further validated with genetic mutations.

The emergence of the genome editing tool CRISPR/Cas9 makes it possible to systematically test tens or hundreds of zebrafish genes for effects on regeneration with tremendous potential for more deeply understanding the differences between mammals and other vertebrates in terms of hearing regeneration. Identification of regeneration-specific genes will not only illuminate the mechanism underlying hair cell regeneration in zebrafish, but also shed light on the design and development of regenerative hearing therapeutics in humans.

Chemical Screening

Chemical screening is an alternative approach to probe the mechanism of hair cell regeneration. It offers several advantages over genetic screening. By being able to control the time window of application, it reveals the requirement of targeted pathways at critical stages of hair cell regeneration. By adjusting chemical concentrations, it allows the researcher to see the effects of partial disruption or activation. In addition, chemical screening can be easily performed on zebrafish larvae [95]. Zebrafish larvae are particularly suitable for chemical screening because large numbers of embryos are easily generated, the small size of the larvae allows the use of multi-well plates, and the simplicity of in vivo staining of lateral line hair cells [96] allows for rapid evaluation of the effects of the compounds. To date, 2 chemical screenings have been conducted using zebrafish larvae to identify small compounds involved in hair cell regeneration [70, 71]. In addition, other chemical screens have focused on identifying compounds that protect hair cells against ototoxins, or identifying compounds with potential ototoxicity [97–103] (fig. 3; table 3). To increase clinical relevance, most screens used ototoxic therapeutics such as neomycin or cisplatin for hair cell ablation, and typically included already FDA-approved drugs in the chemical library for potential clinical repurposing. Although the efficacy of the identified compounds will have to be tested in mammals, the findings from these screens provided valuable information for understanding the molecular mechanisms underlying hair cell regeneration and survival, and potentially provide new therapeutic treatments for both hearing protection and regeneration.

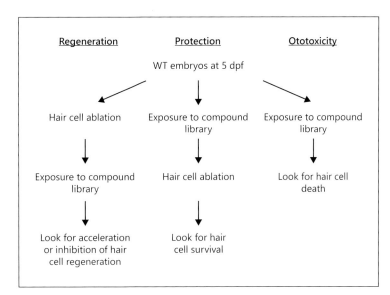

Fig. 3. Flow chart representation of the various forms of chemical screening in zebrafish for regeneration or protection of hearing.

Table 3. Summary of chemical screenings in zebrafish

Goal of screening	Ototoxin	Compounds screened	Source of compounds	Results	Reference
Hair cell regeneration	neomycin	480	470 from Korea Research Institute of Chemical Technology, 10 nature compounds	1 enhancer	[70]
	neomycin	1,680	1,040 from NINDS Custom Collection II, 640 FDA-approved compounds from Enzo Life Sciences	2 enhancers, 6 suppressors	[71]
Hair cell protection	neomycin	10,960	a chemically diverse library	2 protectors	[101]
	neomycin	1,040	NINDS Custom Collection II	7 protectors	[102]
	cisplatin	10,000	ActiProbe 10K (TimTec LLC)	2 protectors	[100]
Hair cell toxicity	N/A	1,040	NINDS Custom Collection II	21 ototoxic	[96]
	N/A	88	anti-cancer drugs (NCI approved ontology drug set)	13 ototoxic	[103]

The Role of Inflammation

Hair cell regeneration is initiated by hair cell ablation. Several studies have shown the involvement of the immune system during regeneration. d'Alencon et al. [104] observed that ablation of neuromast hair cells caused a rapid migration of leukocytes to the sites of injury. Schuck et al. [73] detected differentiated expression of immune response genes MHC classes I and II in the zebrafish inner ear following sound-induced hair cell damage. Namdaran et al. [71] reported that anti-inflammatory agents, dexamethasone and prednisolone, promoted hair cell regeneration.

However, inflammation was shown to stimulate regeneration in other zebrafish tissues such as the brain or the lateral line axon [105, 106]. The relationship between immunity and regeneration is complex, and it will require further studies to clarify the role of immune response in regeneration.

Future Perspectives

Zebrafish has become an important vertebrate organism for modeling human diseases, and its relevance to studies of deafness and hearing regeneration continues to increase as more studies using zebrafish are published. Many large-scale forward and reverse genetic screens utilizing zebrafish have been conducted, and since the completion of the zebrafish genome, the number of molecular tools available for functional genomic studies in zebrafish has rapidly increased. Most of the mutant resources were based on random mutagenesis (retroviral, ENU or transposons) [53–56] that limited our ability to perform systematic functional genomic studies of deafness genes in a targeted manner. With the advent of newer targeted mutagenesis approaches such as CRISPR/Cas9 and TALENs, it is now possible to target a set of genes in a high-throughput and efficient manner [57]. The versatile CRISPR/Cas9 can also target multiple targets simultaneously, which is very useful in inactivating 2 paralogs simultaneously [58].

With the completion of the zebrafish genome and recent advance in genome editing tools, there has never been a better time than now to use zebrafish to model human hearing disorders. It takes much shorter time than before to create zebrafish mutations matching human deafness genes. Studying these zebrafish mutants will lead to a deeper understanding of the functionality of the causative genes of hearing disorders. Thus far, the majority of deafness disease models in zebrafish were based on morpholino-based knock-down or fortuitously identified mutations. With the recent report suggesting that 8/10 morpholino-mediated knockdown phenotypes could not be repeated by their respective genetic mutants [59], moving forward, the emphasis will by necessity be on effects validated by bona fide gene mutations. It will be interesting to see how many zebrafish knockouts of the roughly 100 human deafness genes will recapitulate some or all of the observed human phenotypes. With CRISPR/Cas9, targeting this type of testing is realistic for the first time.

Since the vast majority of hearing loss is associated with aging, the most important question for hearing research is how age affects hair cell survival. We will need more sophisticated tools to tease out roles played by multi-gene phenomena, epigenetics and gene-environment interactions. Zebrafish will be a key model system for complex gene network interactions because it is possible to generate and study enough individual animals to track multiple, small and/or additive genetic or epigenetic effects. Performing such complex associations in mice would be much more difficult purely based on the logistics of generating and caring for the large number of animals needed.

Lastly, because zebrafish are not mammals and still have regenerative capacity after hearing damage, they provide an opportunity to identify potential pathways that could be 'reactivated' in mammals to bring back lost hair cells. Systematic studies to focus researchers on the most promising approaches are underway, and hopefully we will 'hear' of exciting new breakthroughs in the near future.

Acknowledgement

S.M.B. is supported by the Intramural Research Program of the National Human Genome Research Institute, National Institutes of Health. We thank Darryl Leja and Julia Fekecs for their work on figure illustrations.

References

1 Basch ML, Brown RM 2nd, Jen HI, Groves AK: Where hearing starts: the development of the mammalian cochlea. J Anat 2016;228:233–254.

2 Campo P, Morata TC, Hong O: Chemical exposure and hearing loss. Dis Mon 2013;59:119–138.

3 Mittal R, Robalino G, Gerring R, Chan B, Yan D, et al: Immunity genes and susceptibility to otitis media: a comprehensive review. J Genet Genomics 2014;41:567–581.

4 Burchhardt DM, David J, Eckert R, Robinette NL, Carron MA, Zuliani GF: Trauma patterns, symptoms, and complications associated with external auditory canal fractures. Laryngoscope 2015;125:1579–1582.

5 Medina M, Di Lella F, Di Trapani G, Prasad SC, Bacciu A, et al: Cochlear implantation versus auditory brainstem implantation in bilateral total deafness after head trauma: Personal experience and review of the literature. Otol Neurotol 2014;35:260–270.

6 Liu H, Gu Z, Kang HY, Ke X, Shen Y, et al: FCRL3 gene polymorphisms confer risk for sudden sensorineural hearing loss in a Chinese Han population. Gene 2015;570:89–94.

7 Monroe JD, Rajadinakaran G, Smith ME: Sensory hair cell death and regeneration in fishes. Front Cell Neurosci 2015;9:131.

8 Harris JA, Cheng AG, Cunningham LL, MacDonald G, Raible DW, Rubel EW: Neomycin-induced hair cell death and rapid regeneration in the lateral line of zebrafish (Danio rerio). J Assoc Res Otolaryngol 2003;4:219–234.

9 McCauley RD, Fewtrell J, Popper AN: High intensity anthropogenic sound damages fish ears. J Acoust Soc Am 2003;113:638–642.

10 Howe K, Clark MD, Torroja CF, Torrance J, Berthelot C, et al: The zebrafish reference genome sequence and its relationship to the human genome. Nature 2013;496:498–503.

11 Varshney GK, Pei W, LaFave MC, Idol J, Xu L, et al: High-throughput gene targeting and phenotyping in zebrafish using CRISPR/Cas9. Genome Res 2015;25:1030–1042.

12 Atkinson PJ, Huarcaya Najarro E, Sayyid ZN, Cheng AG: Sensory hair cell development and regeneration: similarities and differences. Development 2015;142:1561–1571.

13 Ghysen A, Dambly-Chaudiere C: The lateral line microcosmos. Genes Dev 2007;21:2118–2130.

14 Lush ME, Piotrowski T: Sensory hair cell regeneration in the zebrafish lateral line. Dev Dyn 2014;243:1187–1202.

15 Ma EY, Rubel EW, Raible DW: Notch signaling regulates the extent of hair cell regeneration in the zebrafish lateral line. J Neurosci 2008;28:2261–2273.

16 Nicolson T: The genetics of hearing and balance in zebrafish. Annu Rev Genet 2005;39:9–22.

17 Nicolson T, Rüsch A, Friedrich RW, Granato M, Ruppersberg JP, Nüsslein-Volhard C: Genetic analysis of vertebrate sensory hair cell mechanosensation: the zebrafish circler mutants. Neuron 1998;20:271–283.

18 Whitfield TT, Granato M, van Eeden FJ, Schach U, Brand M, et al: Mutations affecting development of the zebrafish inner ear and lateral line. Development 1996;123:241–254.

19 Granato M, van Eeden FJ, Schach U, Trowe T, Brand M, et al: Genes controlling and mediating locomotion behavior of the zebrafish embryo and larva. Development 1996;123:399–413.

20 Dermitzakis ET, Clark AG: Genetics. Life after GWA studies. Science 2009;326:239–240.

21 Malicki J, Schier AF, Solnica-Krezel L, Stemple DL, Neuhauss SC, et al: Mutations affecting development of the zebrafish ear. Development 1996;123:275–283.

22 Liu XZ, Walsh J, Mburu P, Kendrick-Jones J, Cope MJ, et al: Mutations in the myosin VIIA gene cause non-syndromic recessive deafness. Nat Genet 1997;16:188–190.

23 Luijendijk MW, Van Wijk E, Bischoff AM, Krieger E, Huygen PL, et al: Identification and molecular modelling of a mutation in the motor head domain of myosin VIIA in a family with autosomal dominant hearing impairment (DFNA11). Hum Genet 2004;115:149–156.

24 Riazuddin S, Nazli S, Ahmed ZM, Yang Y, Zulfiqar F, et al: Mutation spectrum of MYO7A and evaluation of a novel nonsyndromic deafness DFNB2 allele with residual function. Hum Mutat 2008;29:502–511.

25 Hildebrand MS, Thorne NP, Bromhead CJ, Kahrizi K, Webster JA, et al: Variable hearing impairment in a DFNB2 family with a novel MYO7A missense mutation. Clin Genet 2010;77:563–571.

26 Weil D, Levy G, Sahly I, Levi-Acobas F, Blanchard S, et al: Human myosin VIIA responsible for the Usher 1B syndrome: a predicted membrane-associated motor protein expressed in developing sensory epithelia. Proc Natl Acad Sci U S A 1996;93:3232–3237.

27 Ernest S, Rauch GJ, Haffter P, Geisler R, Petit C, Nicolson T: Mariner is defective in myosin VIIA: a zebrafish model for human hereditary deafness. Hum Mol Genet 2000;9:2189–2196.

28 Seiler C, Finger-Baier KC, Rinner O, Makhankov YV, Schwarz H, et al: Duplicated genes with split functions: independent roles of protocadherin15 orthologues in zebrafish hearing and vision. Development 2005;132:615–623.

29 Ahmed ZM, Morell RJ, Riazuddin S, Gropman A, Shaukat S, et al: Mutations of MYO6 are associated with recessive deafness, DFNB37. Am J Hum Genet 2003;72:1315–1322.

30 Melchionda S, Ahituv N, Bisceglia L, Sobe T, Glaser F, et al: MYO6, the human homologue of the gene responsible for deafness in snell's waltzer mice, is mutated in autosomal dominant nonsyndromic hearing loss. Am J Hum Genet 2001;69:635–640.

31 Seiler C, Ben-David O, Sidi S, Hendrich O, Rusch A, et al: Myosin VI is required for structural integrity of the apical surface of sensory hair cells in zebrafish. Dev Biol 2004;272:328–338.

32 Sollner C, Rauch GJ, Siemens J, Geisler R, Schuster SC, et al: Mutations in cadherin 23 affect tip links in zebrafish sensory hair cells. Nature 2004;428:955–959.

33 Kazmierczak P, Sakaguchi H, Tokita J, Wilson-Kubalek EM, Milligan RA, et al: Cadherin 23 and protocadherin 15 interact to form tip-link filaments in sensory hair cells. Nature 2007;449:87–91.

34 Ahmed ZM, Riazuddin S, Aye S, Ali RA, Venselaar H, et al: Gene structure and mutant alleles of *PCDH15*: nonsyndromic deafness DFNB23 and type 1 Usher syndrome. Hum Genet 2008;124: 215–223.

35 Ahmed ZM, Riazuddin S, Bernstein SL, Ahmed Z, Khan S, et al: Mutations of the protocadherin gene *PCDH15* cause Usher syndrome type 1F. Am J Hum Genet 2001;69:25–34.

36 Ahmed ZM, Riazuddin S, Ahmad J, Bernstein SL, Guo Y, et al: *PCDH15* is expressed in the neurosensory epithelium of the eye and ear and mutant alleles are responsible for both USH1F and DFNB23. Hum Mol Genet 2003;12: 3215–3223.

37 Van Laer L, Huizing EH, Verstreken M, van Zuijlen D, Wauters JG, et al: Nonsyndromic hearing impairment is associated with a mutation in *DFNA5*. Nat Genet 1998;20:194–197.

38 Busch-Nentwich E, Sollner C, Roehl H, Nicolson T: The deafness gene *dfna5* is crucial for *ugdh* expression and HA production in the developing ear in zebrafish. Development 2004;131:943–951.

39 Peters LM, Anderson DW, Griffith AJ, Grundfast KM, San Agustin TB, et al: Mutation of a transcription factor, *TFCP2L3*, causes progressive autosomal dominant hearing loss, DFNA28. Hum Mol Genet 2002;11:2877–2885.

40 Vona B, Nanda I, Neuner C, Müller T, Haaf T: Confirmation of *GRHL2* as the gene for the DFNA28 locus. Am J Med Genet A 2013;161A:2060–2065.

41 Han Y, Mu Y, Li X, Xu P, Tong J, et al: Grhl2 deficiency impairs otic development and hearing ability in a zebrafish model of the progressive dominant hearing loss DFNA28. Hum Mol Genet 2011;20:3213–3226.

42 Liu F, Yang F, Wen D, Xia W, Hao L, et al: Grhl1 deficiency affects inner ear development in zebrafish. Int J Dev Biol 2015;59:417–423.

43 Naz S, Giguere CM, Kohrman DC, Mitchem KL, Riazuddin S, et al: Mutations in a novel gene, *TMIE*, are associated with hearing loss linked to the *DFNB6* locus. Am J Hum Genet 2002; 71:632–636.

44 Sirmaci A, Ozturkmen-Akay H, Erbek S, Incesulu A, Duman D, et al: A founder *TMIE* mutation is a frequent cause of hearing loss in southeastern Anatolia. Clin Genet 2009;75:562–567.

45 Shen YC, Jeyabalan AK, Wu KL, Hunker KL, Kohrman DC, et al: The transmembrane inner ear (tmie) gene contributes to vestibular and lateral line development and function in the zebrafish (*Danio rerio*). Dev Dyn 2008;237:941–952.

46 Gleason MR, Nagiel A, Jamet S, Vologodskaia M, Lopez-Schier H, Hudspeth AJ: The transmembrane inner ear (Tmie) protein is essential for normal hearing and balance in the zebrafish. Proc Natl Acad Sci U S A 2009;106: 21347–21352.

47 Santos-Cortez RL, Lee K, Giese AP, Ansar M, Amin-Ud-Din M, et al: Adenylate cyclase 1 (*ADCY1*) mutations cause recessive hearing impairment in humans and defects in hair cell function and hearing in zebrafish. Hum Mol Genet 2014;23:3289–3298.

48 Ricci AJ, Fettiplace R: The effects of calcium buffering and cyclic AMP on mechano-electrical transduction in turtle auditory hair cells. J Physiol 1997; 501:111–124.

49 Borck G, Ur Rehman A, Lee K, Pogoda HM, Kakar N, et al: Loss-of-function mutations of *ILDR1* cause autosomal-recessive hearing impairment DFNB42. Am J Hum Genet 2011;88:127–137.

50 Diaz-Horta O, Subasioglu-Uzak A, Grati M, DeSmidt A, Foster J 2nd, et al: FAM65B is a membrane-associated protein of hair cell stereocilia required for hearing. Proc Natl Acad Sci U S A 2014; 111:9864–9868.

51 Gopal SR, Chen DH, Chou SW, Zang J, Neuhauss SC, et al: Zebrafish models for the mechanosensory hair cell dysfunction in Usher syndrome 3 reveal that clarin-1 is an essential hair bundle protein. J Neurosci 2015;35:10188–10201.

52 Phillips JB, Västinsalo H, Wegner J, Clement A, Sankila EM, Westerfield M: The cone-dominant retina and the inner ear of zebrafish express the ortholog of *CLRN1*, the causative gene of human Usher syndrome type 3A. Gene Expr Patterns 2013;13:473–481.

53 Clark KJ, Balciunas D, Pogoda HM, Ding Y, Westcot SE, et al: In vivo protein trapping produces a functional expression codex of the vertebrate proteome. Nat Methods 2011;8:506–515.

54 Kettleborough RN, Busch-Nentwich EM, Harvey SA, Dooley CM, de Bruijn E, et al: A systematic genome-wide analysis of zebrafish protein-coding gene function. Nature 2013;496:494–497.

55 Varshney GK, Huang H, Zhang S, Lu J, Gildea DE, et al: The Zebrafish Insertion Collection (ZInC): a web based, searchable collection of zebrafish mutations generated by DNA insertion. Nucleic Acids Res 2013;41:D861–D864.

56 Varshney GK, Lu J, Gildea DE, Huang H, Pei W, et al: A large-scale zebrafish gene knockout resource for the genome-wide study of gene function. Genome Res 2013;23:727–735.

57 Varshney GK, Burgess SM: Mutagenesis and phenotyping resources in zebrafish for studying development and human disease. Brief Funct Genomics 2014;13: 82–94.

58 Jao LE, Wente SR, Chen W: Efficient multiplex biallelic zebrafish genome editing using a CRISPR nuclease system. Proc Natl Acad Sci U S A 2013;110: 13904–13909.

59 Kok FO, Shin M, Ni CW, Gupta A, Grosse AS, et al: Reverse genetic screening reveals poor correlation between morpholino-induced and mutant phenotypes in zebrafish. Dev Cell 2015;32: 97–108.

60 Brignull HR, Raible DW, Stone JS: Feathers and fins: non-mammalian models for hair cell regeneration. Brain Res 2009;1277:12–23.

61 Rubel EW, Furrer SA, Stone JS: A brief history of hair cell regeneration research and speculations on the future. Hear Res 2013;297:42–51.

62 Lopez-Schier H, Hudspeth AJ: A two-step mechanism underlies the planar polarization of regenerating sensory hair cells. Proc Natl Acad Sci U S A 2006;103: 18615–18620.

63 Mackenzie SM, Raible DW: Proliferative regeneration of zebrafish lateral line hair cells after different ototoxic insults. PLoS One 2012;7:e47257.

64 Roberson DW, Alosi JA, Cotanche DA: Direct transdifferentiation gives rise to the earliest new hair cells in regenerating avian auditory epithelium. J Neurosci Res 2004;78:461–471.

65 Warchol ME: Sensory regeneration in the vertebrate inner ear: differences at the levels of cells and species. Hear Res 2011;273:72–79.

66 Wibowo I, Pinto-Teixeira F, Satou C, Higashijima S, Lopez-Schier H: Compartmentalized Notch signaling sustains epithelial mirror symmetry. Development 2011;138:1143–1152.

67 Behra M, Bradsher J, Sougrat R, Gallardo V, Allende ML, Burgess SM: Phoenix is required for mechanosensory hair cell regeneration in the zebrafish lateral line. PLoS Genet 2009;5:e1000455.

68 Jiang L, Romero-Carvajal A, Haug JS, Seidel CW, Piotrowski T: Gene-expression analysis of hair cell regeneration in the zebrafish lateral line. Proc Natl Acad Sci U S A 2014;111:E1383–E1392.

69 Steiner AB, Kim T, Cabot V, Hudspeth AJ: Dynamic gene expression by putative hair-cell progenitors during regeneration in the zebrafish lateral line. Proc Natl Acad Sci U S A 2014;111:E1393–E1401.

70 Moon IS, So JH, Jung YM, Lee WS, Kim EY, et al: Fucoidan promotes mechanosensory hair cell regeneration following amino glycoside-induced cell death. Hear Res 2011;282:236–242.

71 Namdaran P, Reinhart KE, Owens KN, Raible DW, Rubel EW: Identification of modulators of hair cell regeneration in the zebrafish lateral line. J Neurosci 2012;32:3516–3528.

72 Schuck JB, Smith ME: Cell proliferation follows acoustically-induced hair cell bundle loss in the zebrafish saccule. Hear Res 2009;253:67–76.

73 Schuck JB, Sun H, Penberthy WT, Cooper NG, Li X, Smith ME: Transcriptomic analysis of the zebrafish inner ear points to growth hormone mediated regeneration following acoustic trauma. BMC Neurosci 2011;12:88.

74 Millimaki BB, Sweet EM, Riley BB: Sox2 is required for maintenance and regeneration, but not initial development, of hair cells in the zebrafish inner ear. Dev Biol 2010;338:262–269.

75 Hernandez PP, Olivari FA, Sarrazin AF, Sandoval PC, Allende ML: Regeneration in zebrafish lateral line neuromasts: expression of the neural progenitor cell marker sox2 and proliferation-dependent and-independent mechanisms of hair cell renewal. Dev Neurobiol 2007; 67:637–654.

76 Williams JA, Holder N: Cell turnover in neuromasts of zebrafish larvae. Hear Res 2000;143:171–181.

77 Liang J, Wang D, Renaud G, Wolfsberg TG, Wilson AF, Burgess SM: The *Stat3/Socs3a* pathway is a key regulator of hair cell regeneration in zebrafish. [corrected]. J Neurosci 2012;32:10662–10673.

78 Watt FM: Mammalian skin cell biology: at the interface between laboratory and clinic. Science 2014;346:937–940.

79 Manolio TA, Collins FS, Cox NJ, Goldstein DB, Hindorff LA, et al: Finding the missing heritability of complex diseases. Nature 2009;461:747–753.

80 Feil R, Fraga MF: Epigenetics and the environment: emerging patterns and implications. Nat Rev Genet 2011;13: 97–109.

81 Marshall DJ: Environmentally induced (co)variance in sperm and offspring phenotypes as a source of epigenetic effects. J Exp Biol 2015;218:107–113.

82 Marsit CJ: Influence of environmental exposure on human epigenetic regulation. J Exp Biol 2015;218:71–79.

83 Friedman LM, Dror AA, Mor E, Tenne T, Toren G, et al: MicroRNAs are essential for development and function of inner ear hair cells in vertebrates. Proc Natl Acad Sci U S A 2009;106:7915–7920.

84 Li H, Kloosterman W, Fekete DM: MicroRNA-183 family members regulate sensorineural fates in the inner ear. J Neurosci 2010;30:3254–3263.

85 Rudnicki A, Avraham KB: MicroRNAs: the art of silencing in the ear. EMBO Mol Med 2012;4:849–859.

86 Ushakov K, Rudnicki A, Avraham KB: MicroRNAs in sensorineural diseases of the ear. Front Mol Neurosci 2013;6:52.

87 Lee JH, Daugharthy ER, Scheiman J, Kalhor R, Ferrante TC, et al: Fluorescent in situ sequencing (FISSEQ) of RNA for gene expression profiling in intact cells and tissues. Nat Protoc 2015;10:442–458.

88 Head JR, Gacioch L, Pennisi M, Meyers JR: Activation of canonical Wnt/β-catenin signaling stimulates proliferation in neuromasts in the zebrafish posterior lateral line. Dev Dyn 2013;242: 832–846.

89 Itoh M, Chitnis AB: Expression of proneural and neurogenic genes in the zebrafish lateral line primordium correlates with selection of hair cell fate in neuromasts. Mech Dev 2001;102:263–266.

90 Jacques BE, Montgomery WH 4th, Uribe PM, Yatteau A, Asuncion JD, et al: The role of Wnt/β-catenin signaling in proliferation and regeneration of the developing basilar papilla and lateral line. Dev Neurobiol 2014;74:438–456.

91 Matsuda M, Chitnis AB: Atoh1a expression must be restricted by Notch signaling for effective morphogenesis of the posterior lateral line primordium in zebrafish. Development 2010; 137:3477–3487.

92 Li YH, Chen HY, Li YW, Wu SY, Wangta L, et al: Progranulin regulates zebrafish muscle growth and regeneration through maintaining the pool of myogenic progenitor cells. Sci Rep 2013;3:1176.

93 Mizutari K, Fujioka M, Hosoya M, Bramhall N, Okano HJ, et al: Notch inhibition induces cochlear hair cell regeneration and recovery of hearing after acoustic trauma. Neuron 2013;77: 58–69.

94 He Y, Mei H, Yu H, Sun S, Ni W, Li H: Role of histone deacetylase activity in the developing lateral line neuromast of zebrafish larvae. Exp Mol Med 2014; 46:e94.

95 Gallardo VE, Varshney GK, Lee M, Bupp S, Xu L, et al: Phenotype-driven chemical screening in zebrafish for compounds that inhibit collective cell migration identifies multiple pathways potentially involved in metastatic invasion. Dis Model Mech 2015;8:565–576.

96 Chiu LL, Cunningham LL, Raible DW, Rubel EW, Ou HC: Using the zebrafish lateral line to screen for ototoxicity. J Assoc Res Otolaryngol 2008;9:178–190.

97 Coffin AB, Ou H, Owens KN, Santos F, Simon JA, et al: Chemical screening for hair cell loss and protection in the zebrafish lateral line. Zebrafish 2010;7: 3–11.

98 Esterberg R, Hailey DW, Coffin AB, Raible DW, Rubel EW: Disruption of intracellular calcium regulation is integral to aminoglycoside-induced hair cell death. J Neurosci 2013;33:7513–7525.

99 Ou H, Simon JA, Rubel EW, Raible DW: Screening for chemicals that affect hair cell death and survival in the zebrafish lateral line. Hear Res 2012; 288:58–66.

100 Thomas AJ, Wu P, Raible DW, Rubel EW, Simon JA, Ou HC: Identification of small molecule inhibitors of cisplatin-induced hair cell death: results of a 10,000 compound screen in the zebrafish lateral line. Otol Neurotol 2015;36: 519–525.

101 Owens KN, Santos F, Roberts B, Linbo T, Coffin AB, et al: Identification of genetic and chemical modulators of zebrafish mechanosensory hair cell death. PLoS Genet 2008;4:e1000020.

102 Ou HC, Cunningham LL, Francis SP, Brandon CS, Simon JA, et al: Identification of FDA-approved drugs and bioactives that protect hair cells in the zebrafish (Danio rerio) lateral line and mouse (Mus musculus) utricle. J Assoc Res Otolaryngol 2009;10:191–203.

103 Hirose Y, Simon JA, Ou HC: Hair cell toxicity in anti-cancer drugs: evaluating an anti-cancer drug library for independent and synergistic toxic effects on hair cells using the zebrafish lateral line. J Assoc Res Otolaryngol 2011;12:719–728.

104 d'Alencon CA, Pena OA, Wittmann C, Gallardo VE, Jones RA, et al: A high-throughput chemically induced inflammation assay in zebrafish. BMC Biol 2010;8:151.

105 Kyritsis N, Kizil C, Zocher S, Kroehne V, Kaslin J, et al: Acute inflammation initiates the regenerative response in the adult zebrafish brain. Science 2012;338:1353–1356.

106 Villegas R, Martin SM, O'Donnell KC, Carrillo SA, Sagasti A, Allende ML: Dynamics of degeneration and regeneration in developing zebrafish peripheral axons reveals a requirement for extrinsic cell types. Neural Dev 2012;7:19.

107 van Wijk E, Krieger E, Kemperman MH, De Leenheer EM, Huygen PL, et al: A mutation in the gamma actin 1 (ACTG1) gene causes autosomal dominant hearing loss (DFNA20/26). J Med Genet 2003;40:879–884.

108 Zhu M, Yang T, Wei S, DeWan AT, Morell RJ, et al: Mutations in the gamma-actin gene (ACTG1) are associated with dominant progressive deafness (DFNA20/26). Am J Hum Genet 2003;73:1082–1091.

109 Schrauwen I, Helfmann S, Inagaki A, Predoehl F, Tabatabaiefar MA, et al: A mutation in CABP2, expressed in cochlear hair cells, causes autosomal-recessive hearing impairment. Am J Hum Genet 2012;91:636–645.

110 Modamio-Hoybjor S, Mencia A, Goodyear R, del Castillo I, Richardson G, et al: A mutation in CCDC50, a gene encoding an effector of epidermal growth factor-mediated cell signaling, causes progressive hearing loss. Am J Hum Genet 2007;80:1076–1089.

111 Bork JM, Peters LM, Riazuddin S, Bernstein SL, Ahmed ZM, et al: Usher syndrome 1D and nonsyndromic autosomal recessive deafness DFNB12 are caused by allelic mutations of the novel cadherin-like gene CDH23. Am J Hum Genet 2001;68:26–37.

112 Riazuddin S, Belyantseva IA, Giese AP, Lee K, Indzhykulian AA, et al: Alterations of the CIB2 calcium- and integrin-binding protein cause Usher syndrome type 1J and nonsyndromic deafness DFNB48. Nat Genet 2012;44:1265–1271.

113 Wilcox ER, Burton QL, Naz S, Riazuddin S, Smith TN, et al: Mutations in the gene encoding tight junction claudin-14 cause autosomal recessive deafness DFNB29. Cell 2001;104:165–172.

114 Seco CZ, Oonk AM, Dominguez-Ruiz M, Draaisma JM, Gandia M, et al: Progressive hearing loss and vestibular dysfunction caused by a homozygous nonsense mutation in CLIC5. Eur J Hum Genet 2015;23:189–194.

115 Fransen E, Verstreken M, Verhagen WI, Wuyts FL, Huygen PL, et al: High prevalence of symptoms of Meniere's disease in three families with a mutation in the COCH gene. Hum Mol Genet 1999;8:1425–1429.

116 Hildebrand MS, Tack D, Deluca A, Hur IA, Van Rybroek JM, et al: Mutation in the COCH gene is associated with superior semicircular canal dehiscence. Am J Med Genet A 2009;149A:280–285.

117 Chen W, Kahrizi K, Meyer NC, Riazalhosseini Y, Van Camp G, et al: Mutation of COL11A2 causes autosomal recessive non-syndromic hearing loss at the DFNB53 locus. J Med Genet 2005;42:e61.

118 Abe S, Katagiri T, Saito-Hisaminato A, Usami S, Inoue Y, et al: Identification of CRYM as a candidate responsible for nonsyndromic deafness, through cDNA microarray analysis of human cochlear and vestibular tissues. Am J Hum Genet 2003;72:73–82.

119 Lynch ED, Lee MK, Morrow JE, Welcsh PL, Leon PE, King MC: Nonsyndromic deafness DFNA1 associated with mutation of a human homolog of the Drosophila gene diaphanous. Science 1997;278:1315–1318.

120 Jaworek TJ, Richard EM, Ivanova AA, Giese AP, Choo DI, et al: An alteration in ELMOD3, an Arl2 GTPase-activating protein, is associated with hearing impairment in humans. PLoS Genet 2013;9:e1003774.

121 Behlouli A, Bonnet C, Abdi S, Bouaita A, Lelli A, et al: EPS8, encoding an actin-binding protein of cochlear hair cell stereocilia, is a new causal gene for autosomal recessive profound deafness. Orphanet J Rare Dis 2014;9:55.

122 Naz S, Griffith AJ, Riazuddin S, Hampton LL, Battey JF Jr, et al: Mutations of ESPN cause autosomal recessive deafness and vestibular dysfunction. J Med Genet 2004;41:591–595.

123 Collin RW, Kalay E, Tariq M, Peters T, van der Zwaag B, et al: Mutations of ESRRB encoding estrogen-related receptor beta cause autosomal-recessive nonsyndromic hearing impairment DFNB35. Am J Hum Genet 2008;82:125–138.

124 Wayne S, Robertson NG, DeClau F, Chen N, Verhoeven K, et al: Mutations in the transcriptional activator EYA4 cause late-onset deafness at the DFNA10 locus. Hum Mol Genet 2001;10:195–200.

125 Ain Q, Nazli S, Riazuddin S, Jaleel AU, Riazuddin SA, et al: The autosomal recessive nonsyndromic deafness locus DFNB72 is located on chromosome 19p13.3. Hum Genet 2007;122:445–450.

126 Charizopoulou N, Lelli A, Schraders M, Ray K, Hildebrand MS, et al: Gipc3 mutations associated with audiogenic seizures and sensorineural hearing loss in mouse and human. Nat Commun 2011;2:201.

127 Rehman AU, Gul K, Morell RJ, Lee K, Ahmed ZM, et al: Mutations of GIPC3 cause nonsyndromic hearing loss DFNB72 but not DFNB81 that also maps to chromosome 19p. Hum Genet 2011;130:759–765.

128 Kelsell DP, Dunlop J, Stevens HP, Lench NJ, Liang JN, et al: Connexin 26 mutations in hereditary non-syndromic sensorineural deafness. Nature 1997;387:80–83.

129 Alvarez A, del Castillo I, Villamar M, Aguirre LA, Gonzalez-Neira A, et al: High prevalence of the W24X mutation in the gene encoding connexin-26 (GJB2) in Spanish Romani (gypsies) with autosomal recessive non-syndromic hearing loss. Am J Med Genet A 2005;137A:255–258.

130 Barashkov NA, Dzhemileva LU, Fedorova SA, Teryutin FM, Posukh OL, et al: Autosomal recessive deafness 1A (DFNB1A) in Yakut population isolate in Eastern Siberia: extensive accumulation of the splice site mutation IVS1+1G>A in GJB2 gene as a result of founder effect. J Hum Genet 2011; 56:631–639.

131 Xia JH, Liu CY, Tang BS, Pan Q, Huang L, et al: Mutations in the gene encoding gap junction protein beta-3 associated with autosomal dominant hearing impairment. Nat Genet 1998;20:370–373.

132 del Castillo I, Villamar M, Moreno-Pelayo MA, del Castillo FJ, Alvarez A, et al: A deletion involving the connexin 30 gene in nonsyndromic hearing impairment. New Engl J Med 2002;346:243–249.

133 Walsh T, Shahin H, Elkan-Miller T, Lee MK, Thornton AM, et al: Whole exome sequencing and homozygosity mapping identify mutation in the cell polarity protein GPSM2 as the cause of nonsyndromic hearing loss DFNB82. Am J Hum Genet 2010;87:90–94.

134 Schraders M, Lee K, Oostrik J, Huygen PL, Ali G, et al: Homozygosity mapping reveals mutations of GRXCR1 as a cause of autosomal-recessive non-syndromic hearing impairment. Am J Hum Genet 2010;86:138–147.

135 Imtiaz A, Kohrman DC, Naz S: A frameshift mutation in GRXCR2 causes recessively inherited hearing loss. Hum Mutat 2014;35:618–624.

136 Schultz JM, Khan SN, Ahmed ZM, Riazuddin S, Waryah AM, et al: Noncoding mutations of HGF are associated with nonsyndromic hearing loss, DFNB39. Am J Hum Genet 2009;85:25–39.

137 Santos-Cortez RL, Lee K, Azeem Z, Antonellis PJ, Pollock LM, et al: Mutations in KARS, encoding lysyl-tRNA synthetase, cause autosomal-recessive nonsyndromic hearing impairment DFNB89. Am J Hum Genet 2013;93:132–140.

138 Kubisch C, Schroeder BC, Friedrich T, Lutjohann B, El-Amraoui A, et al: KCNQ4, a novel potassium channel expressed in sensory outer hair cells, is mutated in dominant deafness. Cell 1999;96:437–446.

139 Kalay E, Li Y, Uzumcu A, Uyguner O, Collin RW, et al: Mutations in the lipoma HMGIC fusion partner-like 5 (LHFPL5) gene cause autosomal recessive nonsyndromic hearing loss. Hum Mutat 2006;27:633–639.

140 Longo-Guess CM, Gagnon LH, Cook SA, Wu J, Zheng QY, Johnson KR: A missense mutation in the previously undescribed gene Tmhs underlies deafness in hurry-scurry (hscy) mice. Proc Natl Acad Sci U S A 2005;102:7894–7899.

141 Shabbir MI, Ahmed ZM, Khan SY, Riazuddin S, Waryah AM, et al: Mutations of human TMHS cause recessively inherited non-syndromic hearing loss. J Med Genet 2006;43:634–640.

142 Grillet N, Schwander M, Hildebrand MS, Sczaniecka A, Kolatkar A, et al: Mutations in LOXHD1, an evolutionarily conserved stereociliary protein, disrupt hair cell function in mice and cause progressive hearing loss in humans. Am J Hum Genet 2009;85:328–337.

143 Riazuddin S, Ahmed ZM, Fanning AS, Lagziel A, Kitajiri S, et al: Tricellulin is a tight-junction protein necessary for hearing. Am J Hum Genet 2006;79:1040–1051.

144 Mencia A, Modamio-Hoybjor S, Redshaw N, Morin M, Mayo-Merino F, et al: Mutations in the seed region of human miR-96 are responsible for nonsyndromic progressive hearing loss. Nat Genet 2009;41:609–613.

145 Ahmed ZM, Yousaf R, Lee BC, Khan SN, Lee S, et al: Functional null mutations of MSRB3 encoding methionine sulfoxide reductase are associated with human deafness DFNB74. Am J Hum Genet 2011;88:19–29.

146 Shen X, Liu F, Wang Y, Wang H, Ma J, et al: Down-regulation of msrb3 and destruction of normal auditory system development through hair cell apoptosis in zebrafish. Int J Dev Biol 2015;59:195–203.

147 Donaudy F, Snoeckx R, Pfister M, Zenner HP, Blin N, et al: Nonmuscle myosin heavy-chain gene MYH14 is expressed in cochlea and mutated in patients affected by autosomal dominant hearing impairment (DFNA4). Am J Hum Genet 2004;74:770–776.

148 Lalwani AK, Goldstein JA, Kelley MJ, Luxford W, Castelein CM, Mhatre AN: Human nonsyndromic hereditary deafness DFNA17 is due to a mutation in nonmuscle myosin MYH9. Am J Hum Genet 2000;67:1121–1128.

149 Wang A, Liang Y, Fridell RA, Probst FJ, Wilcox ER, et al: Association of unconventional myosin MYO15 mutations with human nonsyndromic deafness DFNB3. Science 1998;280:1447–1451.

150 Walsh T, Walsh V, Vreugde S, Hertzano R, Shahin H, et al: From flies' eyes to our ears: mutations in a human class III myosin cause progressive nonsyndromic hearing loss DFNB30. Proc Natl Acad Sci U S A 2002;99:7518–7523.

151 Kappler JA, Starr CJ, Chan DK, Kollmar R, Hudspeth AJ: A nonsense mutation in the gene encoding a zebrafish myosin VI isoform causes defects in hair-cell mechanotransduction. Proc Natl Acad Sci U S A 2004;101:13056–13061.

152 Liu XZ, Walsh J, Tamagawa Y, Kitamura K, Nishizawa M, et al: Autosomal dominant non-syndromic deafness caused by a mutation in the myosin VIIA gene. Nat Genet 1997;17:268–269.

153 Wasfy MM, Matsui JI, Miller J, Dowling JE, Perkins BD: Myosin 7aa−/− mutant zebrafish show mild photoreceptor degeneration and reduced electroretinographic responses. Exp Eye Res 2014;122:65–76.

154 Zwaenepoel I, Mustapha M, Leibovici M, Verpy E, Goodyear R, et al: Otoancorin, an inner ear protein restricted to the interface between the apical surface of sensory epithelia and their overlying acellular gels, is defective in autosomal recessive deafness DFNB22. Proc Natl Acad Sci U S A 2002;99:6240–6245.

155 Yasunaga S, Grati M, Cohen-Salmon M, El-Amraoui A, Mustapha M, et al: A mutation in OTOF, encoding otoferlin, a FER-1-like protein, causes DFNB9, a nonsyndromic form of deafness. Nat Genet 1999;21:363–369.

156 Schraders M, Ruiz-Palmero L, Kalay E, Oostrik J, del Castillo FJ, et al: Mutations of the gene encoding otogelin are a cause of autosomal-recessive nonsyndromic moderate hearing impairment. Am J Hum Genet 2012;91:883–889.

157 Chatterjee P, Padmanarayana M, Abdullah N, Holman CL, LaDu J, et al: Otoferlin deficiency in zebrafish results in defects in balance and hearing: rescue of the balance and hearing phenotype with full-length and truncated forms of mouse otoferlin. Mol Cell Biol 2015;35:1043–1054.

158 Yariz KO, Duman D, Seco CZ, Dallman J, Huang M, et al: Mutations in OTOGL, encoding the inner ear protein otogelin-like, cause moderate sensorineural hearing loss. Am J Hum Genet 2012;91:872–882.

159 Yan D, Zhu Y, Walsh T, Xie D, Yuan H, et al: Mutation of the ATP-gated P2X$_2$ receptor leads to progressive hearing loss and increased susceptibility to noise. Proc Natl Acad Sci U S A 2013; 110:2228–2233.

160 Delmaghani S, del Castillo FJ, Michel V, Leibovici M, Aghaie A, et al: Mutations in the gene encoding pejvakin, a newly identified protein of the afferent auditory pathway, cause DFNB59 auditory neuropathy. Nat Genet 2006;38: 770–778.

161 von Ameln S, Wang G, Boulouiz R, Rutherford MA, Smith GM, et al: A mutation in PNPT1, encoding mitochondrial-RNA-import protein PNPase, causes hereditary hearing loss. Am J Hum Genet 2012;91:919–927.

162 de Kok YJ, van der Maarel SM, Bitner-Glindzicz M, Huber I, Monaco AP, et al: Association between X-linked mixed deafness and mutations in the POU domain gene POU3F4. Science 1995;267:685–688.

163 Vahava O, Morell R, Lynch ED, Weiss S, Kagan ME, et al: Mutation in transcription factor POU4F3 associated with inherited progressive hearing loss in humans. Science 1998;279:1950–1954.

164 Liu X, Han D, Li J, Han B, Ouyang X, et al: Loss-of-function mutations in the PRPS1 gene cause a type of nonsyndromic X-linked sensorineural deafness, DFN2. Am J Hum Genet 2010;86: 65–71.

165 Schraders M, Oostrik J, Huygen PL, Strom TM, van Wijk E, et al: Mutations in PTPRQ are a cause of autosomal-recessive nonsyndromic hearing impairment DFNB84 and associated with vestibular dysfunction. Am J Hum Genet 2010;86:604–610.

166 Khan SY, Ahmed ZM, Shabbir MI, Kitajiri S, Kalsoom S, et al: Mutations of the RDX gene cause nonsyndromic hearing loss at the DFNB24 locus. Hum Mutat 2007;28:417–423.

167 Sirmaci A, Erbek S, Price J, Huang M, Duman D, et al: A truncating mutation in SERPINB6 is associated with autosomal-recessive nonsyndromic sensorineural hearing loss. Am J Hum Genet 2010;86:797–804.

168 Mosrati MA, Hammami B, Rebeh IB, Ayadi L, Dhouib L, et al: A novel dominant mutation in SIX1, affecting a highly conserved residue, result in only auditory defects in humans. Eur J Med Genet 2011;54:e484–e488.

169 Ruel J, Emery S, Nouvian R, Bersot T, Amilhon B, et al: Impairment of SLC17A8 encoding vesicular glutamate transporter-3, VGLUT3, underlies nonsyndromic deafness DFNA25 and inner hair cell dysfunction in null mice. Am J Hum Genet 2008;83:278–292.

170 Obholzer N, Wolfson S, Trapani JG, Mo W, Nechiporuk A, et al: Vesicular glutamate transporter 3 is required for synaptic transmission in zebrafish hair cells. J Neurosci 2008;28:2110–2118.

171 Li XC, Everett LA, Lalwani AK, Desmukh D, Friedman TB, et al: A mutation in PDS causes non-syndromic recessive deafness. Nat Genet 1998;18: 215–217.

172 Liu XZ, Ouyang XM, Xia XJ, Zheng J, Pandya A, et al: Prestin, a cochlear motor protein, is defective in non-syndromic hearing loss. Hum Mol Genet 2003;12:1155–1162.

173 Cheng J, Zhu Y, He S, Lu Y, Chen J, et al: Functional mutation of SMAC/DIABLO, encoding a mitochondrial proapoptotic protein, causes human progressive hearing loss DFNA64. Am J Hum Genet 2011;89:56–66.

174 Schraders M, Haas SA, Weegerink NJ, Oostrik J, Hu H, et al: Next-generation sequencing identifies mutations of SMPX, which encodes the small muscle protein, X-linked, as a cause of progressive hearing impairment. Am J Hum Genet 2011;88:628–634.

175 Huebner AK, Gandia M, Frommolt P, Maak A, Wicklein EM, et al: Nonsense mutations in SMPX, encoding a protein responsive to physical force, result in X-chromosomal hearing loss. Am J Hum Genet 2011;88:621–627.

176 Verpy E, Masmoudi S, Zwaenepoel I, Leibovici M, Hutchin TP, et al: Mutations in a new gene encoding a protein of the hair bundle cause non-syndromic deafness at the DFNB16 locus. Nat Genet 2001;29:345–349.

177 Horn HF, Brownstein Z, Lenz DR, Shivatzki S, Dror AA, et al: The LINC complex is essential for hearing. J Clin Invest 2013;123:740–750.

178 Rehman AU, Santos-Cortez RL, Morell RJ, Drummond MC, Ito T, et al: Mutations in TBC1D24, a gene associated with epilepsy, also cause nonsyndromic deafness DFNB86. Am J Hum Genet 2014;94:144–152.

179 Mustapha M, Weil D, Chardenoux S, Elias S, El-Zir E, et al: An alpha-tectorin gene defect causes a newly identified autosomal recessive form of sensorineural pre-lingual non-syndromic deafness, DFNB21. Hum Mol Genet 1999;8:409–412.

180 Verhoeven K, Van Laer L, Kirschhofer K, Legan PK, Hughes DC, et al: Mutations in the human alpha-tectorin gene cause autosomal dominant non-syndromic hearing impairment. Nat Genet 1998;19:60–62.

181 Walsh T, Pierce SB, Lenz DR, Brownstein Z, Dagan-Rosenfeld O, et al: Genomic duplication and overexpression of TJP2/ZO-2 leads to altered expression of apoptosis genes in progressive nonsyndromic hearing loss DFNA51. Am J Hum Genet 2010;87:101–109.

182 Kurima K, Peters LM, Yang Y, Riazuddin S, Ahmed ZM, et al: Dominant and recessive deafness caused by mutations of a novel gene, TMC1, required for cochlear hair-cell function. Nat Genet 2002;30:277–284.

183 Scott HS, Kudoh J, Wattenhofer M, Shibuya K, Berry A, et al: Insertion of beta-satellite repeats identifies a transmembrane protease causing both congenital and childhood onset autosomal recessive deafness. Nat Genet 2001;27: 59–63.

184 Zhao Y, Zhao F, Zong L, Zhang P, Guan L, et al: Exome sequencing and linkage analysis identified tenascin-c (TNC) as a novel causative gene in nonsyndromic hearing loss. PLoS One 2013;8:e69549.

185 Rehman AU, Morell RJ, Belyantseva IA, Khan SY, Boger ET, et al: Targeted capture and next-generation sequencing identifies C9orf75, encoding taperin, as the mutated gene in nonsyndromic deafness DFNB79. Am J Hum Genet 2010;86:378–388.

186 Li Y, Pohl E, Boulouiz R, Schraders M, Nurnberg G, et al: Mutations in TPRN cause a progressive form of autosomal-recessive nonsyndromic hearing loss. Am J Hum Genet 2010;86:479–484.

187 Shahin H, Walsh T, Sobe T, Abu Sa'ed J, Abu Rayan A, et al: Mutations in a novel isoform of TRIOBP that encodes a filamentous-actin binding protein are responsible for DFNB28 recessive nonsyndromic hearing loss. Am J Hum Genet 2006;78:144–152.

188 Riazuddin S, Khan SN, Ahmed ZM, Ghosh M, Caution K, et al: Mutations in TRIOBP, which encodes a putative cytoskeletal-organizing protein, are associated with nonsyndromic recessive deafness. Am J Hum Genet 2006; 78:137–143.

189 Delmaghani S, Aghaie A, Michalski N, Bonnet C, Weil D, Petit C: Defect in the gene encoding the EAR/EPTP domain-containing protein TSPEAR causes DFNB98 profound deafness. Hum Mol Genet 2012;21:3835–3844.

190 Ouyang XM, Xia XJ, Verpy E, Du LL, Pandya A, et al: Mutations in the alternatively spliced exons of USH1C cause non-syndromic recessive deafness. Hum Genet 2002;111:26–30.

191 Ahmed ZM, Smith TN, Riazuddin S, Makishima T, Ghosh M, et al: Nonsyndromic recessive deafness DFNB18 and Usher syndrome type IC are allelic mutations of USHIC. Hum Genet 2002;110:527–531.

192 Bespalova IN, Van Camp G, Bom SJ, Brown DJ, Cryns K, et al: Mutations in the Wolfram syndrome 1 gene (WFS1) are a common cause of low frequency sensorineural hearing loss. Hum Mol Genet 2001;10:2501–2508.

193 Young TL, Ives E, Lynch E, Person R, et al: Non-syndromic progressive hearing loss DFNA38 is caused by heterozygous missense mutation in the Wolfram syndrome gene WFS1. Hum Mol Genet 2001;10:2509–2514.

194 Mburu P, Mustapha M, Varela A, Weil D, El-Amraoui A, et al: Defects in whirlin, a PDZ domain molecule involved in stereocilia elongation, cause deafness in the whirler mouse and families with DFNB31. Nat Genet 2003;34:421–428.

Shawn M. Burgess, PhD
Translational and Functional Genomics Branch
National Human Genome Research Institute
National Institutes of Health
9000 Rockville Pike
Bethesda, MD 20892 (USA)
E-Mail burgess@mail.nih.gov

Vona B, Haaf T (eds): Genetics of Deafness. Monogr Hum Genet. Basel, Karger, 2016, vol 20, pp 132–141
(DOI: 10.1159/000444570)

Current Understanding and Potential of Gene Therapy for Hearing Restoration in Humans

Omar Akil[a] · Lawrence Lustig[b]

[a]Department of Otolaryngology – Head and Neck Surgery, University of California, San Francisco, Calif., and [b]Department of Otolaryngology – Head and Neck Surgery, Columbia University Medical Center, New York, N.Y., USA

Abstract

Genetic forms of sensorineural deafness account for almost half of all patients with congenital hearing loss (HL). Increasing knowledge of the underlying molecular and genetic mechanisms that lead to HL raises the possibility for novel therapeutics, such as those based on gene transfer and related methods that influence gene expression in affected tissues. Over the past decade, there has been renewed interest in cochlear gene therapy for the treatment of a variety of causes of HL. The last several years have seen significant advances in gene therapy for HL in mouse models of deafness that further supports the promise of gene therapy approaches to improving hearing health. These studies document that both replacing an absent gene and downregulating a dominant mutated gene can restore hearing. It is thus reasonable to predict that the successful treatment approaches increasingly being reported in mouse models of HL will establish a framework for developing gene replacement therapies in humans. Here, we review the most recent advances in cochlear gene therapy. This review will cover the animal models used in these studies, the most widely employed viral vectors, potential routes of delivery into the inner ear, and an overview of several genetic deficiencies in mouse models that have been successfully addressed. Lastly, this review elaborates on research directed towards spiral ganglion neuronal preservation and regeneration.

© 2016 S. Karger AG, Basel

Introduction and an Overview of the Ear

The inner ear is a complex structure that enables sound to be perceived by the brain. In order for the ear to accomplish this feat, 2 fundamental processes need to occur. Initially, sound must be broken down into its component frequencies and spread along the length of the inner ear. Then, at each of these locations, the motion induced by the sound waves must be converted into an electric impulse to be transmitted to the brain. Critical to this concept is what is referred to as the 'tonotopicity' of the inner ear – each location of the organ of Corti corresponds to a graded, unique frequency, similar to that of a piano keyboard. This is achieved in a remarkably elegant solution.

Initially, sound travels down the external auditory canal to the tympanic membrane. Sound processing occurs even at this early passive stage, with the structure of the auricle and canal preferentially amplifying sounds in the human auditory speech frequency range. The tympanic membrane is coupled to the malleus, the first of the 3 ossicles. The sound waves travel from the tympanic membrane and malleus through the 2nd and 3rd ossicles, the incus and stapes, respectively, to reach the inner ear. The relative size of the tympanic membrane compared to the base of the stapes (oval window), combined with the lever-like action of the ossicles, results in an ~30:1 amplification of sound energy, allowing the sound impulse to overcome the air (middle ear)-fluid (inner ear) interface. Once in the inner ear, the fluid waves travel through parallel curved chambers, the scala vestibuli and scala tympani. The relative pressure difference between these 2 scalae causes motion of the 3rd scala (scala media), sandwiched between these, to move. Within the scala media lies the organ of Corti. Thus, motion is transmitted to the organ of Corti by the movement of the fluid waves within the surrounding scalae. The physical structure of the organ of Corti naturally parses sound along the basilar membrane of the scala media in a 'tonotopic' manner, such that high frequency sounds preferentially cause motion at one end of the organ of Corti, while low frequencies result in motion at the other end, due to the physical structure of the basilar membrane upon which the organ of Corti is sitting. This is generally how the ear achieves the first goal of sound processing – separating sound into its fundamental frequencies along the length of the organ of Corti.

The organ of Corti is the critical structure that achieves the second aim of sound processing – conversion of the sound energy to an electrical signal of the auditory nerve. At each location along the organ of Corti there are inner hair cells (so named because stereocilia tips that project from their apical surface resemble hairs) that move in response to motion induced by sound pressure differences of the scalae. As this motion occurs, the stereocilia tips, embedded in the tectorial membrane, are physically bent. This deflection opens a spring-gated ion channel allowing positively charged ions to enter the hair cell. This inward current ultimately results in the release of neurotransmitter at the base of the inner hair cell, which in turn depolarizes the primary afferent auditory neuron synapsing at the base of that hair cell. From there, the auditory signal is transmitted through several orders of neurons within the brainstem and midbrain, with processing at each stage, and ultimately to the auditory cortex.

While a majority of the incoming auditory signal occurs in this manner, there is an efferent feedback mechanism that allows the ear to modify the incoming signal. This is accomplished through the outer hair cells in the organ of Corti, which receive the majority of outgoing, efferent auditory neurons. The role of the efferent auditory system and outer hair cells is to provide fine-tuning of the incoming auditory signal, increase frequency discrimination as well as provide protection against noise-induced hearing loss (HL).

In this highly tuned and extraordinarily sensitive system, it is no coincidence that a number of genetic abnormalities along the auditory transduction pathway have been described. Abnormalities at any location along the auditory transduction pathway, from the ear canal to the auditory nerve, can cause HL. Overall, hearing impairment is the most common sensory deficit in humans [1]. Approximately 1.5 in 1,000 newborns suffer from congenital hearing impairment [2], and genetic forms of sensorineural deafness account for almost half of all patients with HL [3]. Treatment options for inherited forms of deafness are quite limited, consisting only of hearing amplification for mild to severe HL, and cochlear implantation for severe to profound HL [1, 4]. These treatments, though quite beneficial for those who receive these technologies, still have great limitations and do not restore hearing to normal levels [1]. For these reasons, cochlear gene therapy has been suggested as an alternative treatment for both genetic and acquired forms of HL.

Application of gene replacement therapy towards the treatment of deafness holds promise for several reasons. Foremost, there are large numbers of single-gene defects that lead to sensorineural HL. Further, vectors have the ability to target specific cells in which these genes manifest their function, including hair cells and spiral ganglion neurons. In theory, the introduction of the normal (wild-type) gene into these cells should be able to restore function or prevent the degradation, and subsequent HL, that would otherwise occur. Thus, unlike currently available technologies, gene therapy has the potential to restore normal, or near normal auditory function, reversing the adverse effects of genetic disease.

Animal Models

There are a number of animal models used in auditory research, from cats to primates to gerbils. However, the mouse remains the most important for studying gene therapy for a variety of reasons. While the small size of mouse cochleae does present some surgical difficulties, mice are relatively easy to work with and maintain, cost-efficient, and have relatively high reproduction rates, with several experimental advantages over other species [5]. All auditory structures present in the human ear exist in the mouse [6]. Additionally, the mouse genome is the most characterized of all mammalian organisms [6]. Extensive genetic studies in mice combined with technological advances have made it possible to generate genetically modified mice in a reproducible way across laboratories [7–11]. The availability of a number of mutant mice (e.g. shaker-1 and Snell's walter), with well-characterized inherited HL analogous

to human auditory dysfunction, and the fact that mice and humans share 99% of their genes [12], makes mice uniquely suitable for molecular manipulations [6, 13, 14]. Thus, correcting hearing using virally mediated gene therapy in a mouse model for human deafness is an appropriate and necessary first step in the search for a cure for human disease.

Viral Vectors

With an understanding of the genes used in cochlear gene therapy, it is important to consider the vector as it has a direct and essential impact upon the successful delivery of a targeted gene. There are several viruses that have been investigated for cochlear gene delivery, though the two that have received the most attention are adenovirus (AV) and adeno-associated virus (AAV). The advantage of AV is its ability to carry large genes, to produce high functional titers, and to transfect both dividing and non-dividing cells [15]. The principle disadvantage, particularly as it relates to genetic deafness, is the transient nature of transgene expression of AV vectors, often limited to weeks [16].

For genetic deafness, AAV is currently the vector with the most potential promise. AAV are replication-deficient viruses and can efficiently transfer the transgene to a number of different cochlear cell types, including non-replicating neurons and hair cells [17]. Because AAV entry into the cell is mediated by specific receptors [18], different AAV subtypes can have a direct effect on the cells able to be transfected. AAV can very effectively transduce inner hair cells [17, 19], where a number of genetic deficiencies are focused, but less so outer hair cells. Another advantage of AAV is that they can incorporate into the host genome resulting in stable, long-term expression of the transgene [20]. Since long-term expression is very important for stable rescue of genetic defects, this becomes a critical advantage over a vector such as AV, which only provides transgene expression for up to several weeks. AAV has also been shown to be safe and effective in several clinical trials. Because AAV are not associated with any human disease or infection and demonstrate no ototoxicity [21–23], they remain the ideal candidate for use in gene therapy for inherited forms of HL [24].

The biggest limitation of AAV as a vector for gene therapy is its relatively small packaging capacity, allowing only ~5 kb of DNA as an insert, and many of the genes known to cause HL are larger than 5 kb. However, recent advances have opened the door to potentially allowing AAV to shuttle larger inserts into host cells. One recent study by Dyka et al. [25] used a 'dual vector' approach, splitting the desired gene into 2 different inserts, each containing an overlapping sequence that could individually fit into 2 separate AAV vectors. Once a cell was dually-infected with both AAV constructs, the overlapping sequences on each DNA insert recombined, allowing the full cDNA to reform. This approach was used to successfully express the myosin VIIA gene (~6.7 kb) in vitro and in vivo with high efficiency and 100% fidelity to the predicted sequence [25]. Using this dual vector approach, it is thus potentially possible to use AAV for delivery of genes up to 10 kb in size, greatly increasing the number of potential targets of genetic HL.

Methods of Gene Delivery

There are 3 principle methods of delivering genes (and other substances) into the cochlea: round window membrane (RWM) diffusion, RWM injection, and cochleostomy. There are potential advantages and disadvantages of each of these approaches [26]. The primary goal with these methodologies is the safe administration of the vector-transgene complex into the cochlea with minimal damage and maximal transgene expression [27]. While there are studies describing

RWM diffusion, in general the round window does not efficiently transport the vector across without a manipulation such as enzymatic digestion or use of hyaluronic acid [28, 29]. Thus, cochleostomy or RWM injection are the preferred routes. Akil et al. [30] attempted both methods in their study of viral delivery into the cochlea and found that RWM delivery was more efficient in restoring hearing in mice lacking VGLUT3 than the cochleostomy technique. Askew et al. [31] applied a similar RWM approach in their successful transfection of cochlea in TMC1-deficient mice. In addition, the cochleostomy has been characterized as being technically more challenging to perform, and it is associated with localized trauma and inflammation [27]. In contrast, the post-auricular method can easily be performed in mice and has experimentally shown that the percentage of mice recovering hearing is much higher via direct injection of the virus through the RWM than with viral delivery via cochleostomy [30, 32].

Many other studies describe the post-auricular surgical approach as the ideal method for cochlear gene therapy in laboratory animals [32–35]. This surgical approach involves negligible or no damage to essential structures of the inner and middle ear while completely preserving hearing. This post-auricular technique demonstrated successful transgene expression within the inner hair cells, outer hair cells and supporting cells, as well as high transduction rates [30]. Recently, it appears that the post-auricular approach is more commonly used than other methods because it enables rapid and direct delivery into the scala tympani while minimizing blood loss and avoiding animal mortality [32]. Currently, hearing preserving cochlear implantation in humans can be accomplished via a RWM approach or cochleostomy, though the RWM approach is more widely practiced [36]. Further, the RWM in humans can often be visualized through a transcanal procedure, ideal for future human gene therapy applications, since this would limit the morbidity of delivery. These advantages make the RWM approach a promising and ideal candidate method of cochlear gene therapy in possible future human applications.

Cochlear Gene Therapy Successes in Animal Models of Genetic Deafness

Connexin 26 – GJB2

Mutations in the Connexin 26 (Cx26) gene, which codes for gap junctions, account for a large percentage of cases of genetic deafness, and *GJB2* remains one of the most important targets of gene therapy for HL [37]. Given the widespread localization of gap junctions within the cochlea, however, it is also one of the most challenging targets, since all cell types expressing gap junctions would need to be transduced in order to prevent HL. One challenge studying Cx26 is that a germline mutation results in death in utero. Thus, the models that have been created involve some form of postnatal genetic manipulation. One early study by Maeda et al. [38] employed a small interfering RNA (siRNA) approach in a dominant-negative mutation of the *Gjb2* gene, which encodes Cx26. In this study, the dominant-negative mutation, when delivered to the ear, caused HL. Introduction of siRNA against the mutant gene was subsequently able to knock-down the exogenously delivered mutant and prevent the HL. A more recent study involved a conditional knockout mouse [39]. In this study, AAV delivery of Cx26 resulted in widespread expression of the connexin 26 protein, as well as reduced cell death and spiral ganglion neuronal degeneration. However, the hearing, as measured by acoustic brainstem response (ABR) thresholds, was not substantially improved as compared to untreated mice. Together, these important studies on Cx26 showed that manipulation of a mutant protein can be achieved without compromising optimal levels of the normal protein, a critical requirement for successful translation of this approach to humans.

Vesicular Glutamate Transporter 3 (VGLUT3/ SLC17A8)

A missense mutation in the human *SLC17A8* gene has been shown to be responsible for a progressive high frequency HL seen in human DFNA25 [40]. In the ear, VGLUT3 localizes to the inner hair cells, and a transgenic mouse lacking VGLUT3 was shown to be deaf at birth due to loss of glutamate transmission [41]. Other than changes at the ribbon synapse and loss of hearing, all other morphological features of the ear were intact, including outer hair cell function, making this a potentially useful target for a cochlear gene therapy approach.

Using AAV1, Akil et al. [30] delivered the VGLUT3 gene to the ear using several techniques. In these studies, hearing in the knockout mice was restored to normal ABR threshold levels, while many of the physiologic and anatomic changes were reversed with this treatment. While the VGLUT3 mouse model was different from the human nonsyndromic HL (missense mutation in the human vs. null-mutation in the mouse), the successful approach nonetheless provided a strong proof of principle that single-gene defects that lead to HL could be effectively treated with a gene therapy approach and represented an important milestone.

TMC1

TMC1 is a gene integral to hair cell function and believed to be involved in the transduction channel [42]. Mice lacking or having mutations in TMC1 have disorders of hearing and balance, and are models for both autosomal dominant and recessive forms of HL in humans and are responsible for as many as 8% of cases of genetic deafness [43, 44].

In a recent study, Askew et al. [31], employing a technique similar to Akil et al. [30], used AAV2/1 to transfect TMC1-deficient mice. The group showed very robust transfection of inner hair cells but limited outer hair cell transfection. Functionally, the mice had restoration of ABR thresholds and restoration of electrophysiologic transduction, but no restoration of efferent function, as would be predicted based on a lack of outer hair cell transfection. In this important study, by advancing the findings of Akil et al. [30], the group has shown that rescue of auditory function in a clinically relevant mouse models of human deafness is feasible. However, the lack of outer hair cell transfection and restoration of the efferent system is an important limitation that will one day need to be overcome in order to translate this into humans.

Usher 1C

An alternate approach was described by Lentz et al. [45]. Using a mouse model of Usher syndrome type 1C, a form of hereditary deafness and blindness, the investigators used antisense oligonucleotides to correct defective pre-mRNA splicing of transcripts from the mutated gene, resulting in increased protein expression, improved stereocilia organization in the cochlea, and rescue of cochlear hair cells, vestibular function and hearing in mice. This study is important on several levels. The nature of the mutation in Usher syndrome leads to a progressive degeneration of the sensory hair cells of the cochlea, and the antisense RNA treatment delays or prevents that degeneration, preserving hair cell function. There are many similar genetic defects that also lead to a progressive degeneration of the sensory cells of the cochlea, and this study provides hope that many of these genetic defects can be treated in a similar fashion.

All these results document that genetic causes of deafness can be treated in animal models mimicking human disease, and argue for future clinical trials once details such as vector choice and delivery method, timing of delivery, and promoter design can be optimized. In a similar vein, there are a number of important advances in cellular regeneration and stem cell therapies for cochlear regeneration that is beyond the scope of this review. However, it is important to note that breakthroughs in cellular regeneration may not benefit those with genetic deafness, since the underlying genetic background remains unchanged with these therapies [46, 47]. Thus, the cochlea continues to be an attractive target for gene therapy due to the relative ease of access and confinement of its fluid spaces, and potential for long-term changes to the genetic background to cure HL [46, 47].

Other Potential Genes of Interest

Genetic defects play a significant role in sensorineural HL, one of the most common neurological disorders. Hereditary hearing impairment genes whose dysfunction or mutation is associated with HL represent a potential subset of targets for gene therapy. Potential applications include the correction of genetic forms of HL with the expression of the wild-type form of the mutant deafness genes or the introduction of growth factors to enhance spiral ganglion cell survival.

To date, 75 different deafness genes have been identified, and each could represent a potential target for gene therapy. Several of these genes are associated with Usher syndrome and hair cell cytoarchitecture including *MYO7A*, *USH1C*, *CDH23*, *MYO6*, *MYO15A*, *KCNQ1*, and *KCNE1* [48]. The promising results from the work by Lentz et al. [45] and Askew et al. [31] suggest that some of these targets could be treated in a similar fashion. Some of the other more common forms of hereditary deafness, such as those caused by the most relevant forms of connexin gene mutation which collectively account for more than a half of all cases of human hereditary deafness [37], also present attractive potential targets. Beyond connexins, one study by Kesser et al. [49] evaluated the potassium channel KCNQ4, defective in the deafness seen in DFNA2, an isolated autosomal-dominant form of deafness. The authors demonstrated that AV-mediated delivery of *KCNQ4* can transduce cultured human vestibular tissue. However, this work has not yet been translated into an animal model. In summary, only a small number

Table 1. Cochlear gene therapy in animal models of human deafness

Reference	Human hearing loss	Gene	Animal model	Vector	Promoter
Maeda et al., 2005 [38]	DFNA3, DFNB1	*GJB2*-connexin 26	WT mouse	liposome-siRNA	
Yu et al., 2014 [39]	DFNA3, DFNB1	*GJB2*-connexin 26	conditional KO mouse	AAV2/1	CB7
Akil et al., 2012 [30]	DFNA25	*VGLUT3*	VGLUT3 KO mouse	AAV1	CBA
Askew et al., 2015 [31]	DFNB7/11, DFNA36	*TMC1*	TMC1 KO mouse	AAV2/1	CBA
Lentz et al., 2013 [45]	Usher 1C	*USH1C*	216AA transgenic mouse	ASO	

AAV = Adeno-associated virus; ASO = antisense oligonucleotide; KO = knockout; siRNA = small interfering RNA; WT = wild type.

of genes, in which defects have been shown to lead to sensorineural HL in humans, have been studied using gene therapy techniques in animal models (table 1). Given these promising early results in mouse models of these mutations, it is anticipated that many more studies in other models of human deafness will follow soon.

Spiral Ganglion Neuronal Preservation and Regeneration

One additional important application of cochlear gene therapy beyond that for genetic forms of HL concerns itself with spiral ganglion neuronal preservation or regeneration. Primary or secondary loss of spiral ganglion neurons is a well-known cause of sensorineural HL in humans. Spiral ganglion neurons can degenerate as a consequence of mechanical stress, toxic insults, and ischemia, among others causes. Spiral ganglion neurons are also critical for the function of cochlear implants, as the primary afferent neuronal population being stimulated by the device. Thus, methods of either preserving or regenerating spiral ganglion neurons have become of great interest to basic science and translational researchers, either to preserve native hearing, or improve the function of cochlear implants. Survival of neurons in the cochlea is dependent on a delicate balance of neurotrophic factors and calcium influx elicited

by depolarization. A number of studies have shown that glial cell-derived neurotrophic factor (GDNF), brain-derived neurotrophic factor (BDNF) and neurotrophin-3 (NT-3) are all capable of rescuing neurons following insult [50–53]. Intracochlear injection or expression of neurotrophic factors further improves spiral ganglion neuronal survival. Several studies have demonstrated that the preservation of spiral ganglion neurons can potentially benefit from cochlear gene therapy. Wise et al. [54] used AAV-mediated transduction of BDNF and NT-3 in animals deafened for up to 8 weeks prior to viral delivery. What is significant is that the authors showed that viral transduction of cells was possible even after severe degeneration of the organ of Corti [54]. In addition, Wise et al. [54] noted a great increase in spiral ganglion survival in the entire basal turn for cochleae that received gene therapy compared to controls. Another study using AAV-mediated delivery of BDNF by Shibata et al. [55] demonstrated that the forced expression of BDNF in mesothelial or epithelial cells in deafened guinea pigs induced regrowth of nerve fibers towards the cells that secrete the neurotrophin. Moreover, the authors indicated that this neuronal regeneration was accompanied by a preservation of spiral ganglion neurons. A third recent study used AV-mediated human B-nerve growth factor (Ad-hNGFB) gene transfer for HL in rats [56]. Wu et al. [56] demonstrated that the ABR threshold shifts in the NGFB-transduced group were significantly smaller than those of non-transduced controls. Finally, and of significance, the authors revealed that the spiral ganglion count in the transduced group was significantly greater than that of the non-transduced controls [56]. These studies illustrate that potential applications of cochlear gene therapy go beyond genetic deafness, and suggest it to be a promising candidate for a number of future human applications.

Conclusion

In recent years, a large and ever increasing number of genes whose mutations lead to human deafness have been identified. Knowledge of the underlying molecular genetic mechanisms that cause HL raises the possibility for novel therapeutics, such as those based on cochlear gene therapy that influence gene expression in affected tissues. Several technical advances have been made in translational cochlear gene therapy studies that put us closer to seeing successful application in humans. A recently begun US FDA

(Food and Drug Administration) trial of gene therapy for acquired HL using the atonal 1 gene to attempt hair cell regeneration in humans is a testament to these advances. This human clinical study is the result of a number of basic and translational scientific studies that have shown that the *ATOH1* gene (also termed *Math1* in mice and *HATH1* in humans) is responsible for causing supporting cells of the inner ear to terminally differentiate into auditory hair cells, and transfecting animals with an AV containing the *Math1* gene results in new auditory hair cells with functional hearing and balance recovery [23, 35, 46, 47]. Results from this clinical trial, the first human cochlear gene therapy study attempted, will likely yield valuable data that will influence future gene therapy trials for genetic forms of HL. Ultimately however, successful treatment of genetic HL using gene therapy will require parallel advances in genetic testing, a thorough understanding of the correlation between genotype and phenotype, and advances in vector design and delivery. However, the field has reached a stage where those advances no longer seem to be insurmountable.

References

1 Kral A, O'Donoghue GM: Profound deafness in childhood. N Engl J Med 2010;363:1438–1450.

2 Di Domenico M, Ricciardi C, Martone T, Mazzarella N, Cassandro C, et al: Towards gene therapy for deafness. J Cell Physiol 2011;226:2494–2499.

3 Shearer AE, Hildebrand MS, Sloan CM, Smith RJ: Deafness in the genomics era. Hear Res 2011;282:1–9.

4 Petersen MB, Willems PJ: Non-syndromic, autosomal-recessive deafness. Clin Genet 2006;69:371–392.

5 Friedman LM, Dror AA, Avraham KB: Mouse models to study inner ear development and hereditary hearing loss. Int J Dev Biol 2007;51:609–631.

6 Jero J, Tseng CJ, Mhatre AN, Lalwani AK: A surgical approach appropriate for targeted cochlear gene therapy in the mouse. Hear Res 2001;151:106–114.

7 Chang EH, Van Camp G, Smith RJ: The role of connexins in human disease. Ear Hear 2003;24:314–323.

8 Cohen-Salmon M, Ott T, Michel V, Hardelin JP, Perfettini I, et al: Targeted ablation of connexin26 in the inner ear epithelial gap junction network causes hearing impairment and cell death. Curr Biol 2002;12:1106–1111.

9 Nickel R, Forge A: Gap junctions and connexins in the inner ear: their roles in homeostasis and deafness. Curr Opin Otolaryngol Head Neck Surg 2008;16: 452–457.

10 Lv P, Wei D, Yamoah EN: Kv7-type channel currents in spiral ganglion neurons: involvement in sensorineural hearing loss. J Biol Chem 2010;285: 34699–34707.

11 Leibovici M, Safieddine S, Petit C: Mouse models for human hereditary deafness. Curr Top Dev Biol 2008;84: 385–429.

12 Rosenthal N, Brown S: The mouse ascending: perspectives for human-disease models. Nat Cell Biol 2007;9:993–999.

13 Dror AA, Avraham KB: Hearing loss: mechanisms revealed by genetics and cell biology. Annu Rev Genet 2009;43: 411–437.

14 Richardson GP, de Monvel JB, Petit C: How the genetics of deafness illuminates auditory physiology. Annu Rev Physiol 2011;73:311–334.

15 Campos SK, Barry MA: Current advances and future challenges in adenoviral vector biology and targeting. Curr Gene Ther 2007;7:189–204.

16 Lentz TB, Gray SJ, Samulski RJ: Viral vectors for gene delivery to the central nervous system. Neurobiol Dis 2012;48:179–188.

17 Kilpatrick LA, Li Q, Yang J, Goddard JC, Fekete DM, Lang H: Adeno-associated virus-mediated gene delivery into the scala media of the normal and deafened adult mouse ear. Gene Ther 2011;18:569–578.

18 Nam HJ, Lane MD, Padron E, Gurda B, McKenna R, et al: Structure of adeno-associated virus serotype 8, a gene therapy vector. J Virol 2007;81:12260–12271.

19 Ryan AF, Mullen LM, Doherty JK: Cellular targeting for cochlear gene therapy. Adv Otorhinolaryngol 2009;66:99–115.

20 Xia L, Yin S, Wang J: Inner ear gene transfection in neonatal mice using adeno-associated viral vector: a comparison of two approaches. PLoS One 2012;7:e43218.

21 Husseman J, Raphael Y: Gene therapy in the inner ear using adenovirus vectors. Adv Otorhinolaryngol 2009;66:37–51.

22 Ballana E, Wang J, Venail F, Estivill X, Puel JL, et al: Efficient and specific transduction of cochlear supporting cells by adeno-associated virus serotype 5. Neurosci Lett 2008;442:134–139.

23 Praetorius M, Brough DE, Hsu C, Plinkert PK, Pfannenstiel SC, Staecker H: Adenoviral vectors for improved gene delivery to the inner ear. Hear Res 2009;248:31–38.

24 Kay MA, Glorioso CG, Naldini L: Viral vectors for gene therapy: the art of turning infectious agents into vehicles of therapeutics. Nat Med 2001;7:33–40.

25 Dyka FM, Boye SL, Chiodo VA, Hauswirth WW, Boye SE: Dual adeno-associated virus vectors result in efficient in vitro and in vivo expression of an oversized gene *MYO7A*. Hum Gene Ther Methods 2014;25:166–177.

26 Kesser BW, Lalwani AK: Gene therapy and stem cell transplantation: strategies for hearing restoration. Adv Otorhinolaryngol 2009;66:64–86.

27 Jero J, Mhatre AN, Tseng CJ, Stern RE, Coling DE, et al: Cochlear gene delivery through an intact round window membrane in mouse. Hum Gene Ther 2001;12:539–548.

28 Shibata SB, Cortez SR, Wiler JA, Swiderski DL, Raphael Y: Hyaluronic acid enhances gene delivery into the cochlea. Hum Gene Ther 2012;23:302–310.

29 Wang H, Murphy R, Taaffe D, Yin S, Xia L, et al: Efficient cochlear gene transfection in guinea-pigs with adeno-associated viral vectors by partial digestion of round window membrane. Gene Ther 2012;19:255–263.

30 Akil O, Seal RP, Burke K, Wang C, Alemi A, et al: Restoration of hearing in the VGLUT3 knockout mouse using virally-mediated gene therapy. Neuron 2012;75:283–293.

31 Askew C, Rochat C, Pan B, Asai Y, Ahmed H, et al: *Tmc* gene therapy restores auditory function in deaf mice. Sci Transl Med 2015;7:295ra108.

32 Akil O, Rouse SL, Chan DK, Lustig LR: Surgical method for virally mediated gene delivery to the mouse inner ear through the round window membrane. J Vis Exp 2015;97:e52187.

33 Carvalho GJ, Lalwani AK: The effect of cochleostomy and intracochlear infusion on auditory brain stem response threshold in the guinea pig. Am J Otol 1999;20:87–90.

34 Kawamoto K, Oh SH, Kanzaki S, Brown N, Raphael Y: The functional and structural outcome of inner ear gene transfer via the vestibular and cochlear fluids in mice. Mol Ther 2001;4:575–585.

35 Praetorius M, Baker K, Weich CM, Plinkert PK, Staecker H: Hearing preservation after inner ear gene therapy: the effect of vector and surgical approach. ORL J Otorhinolaryngol Relat Spec 2003;65:211–214.

36 Friedland DR, Runge-Samuelson C: Soft cochlear implantation: rationale for the surgical approach. Trends Amplif 2009;13:124–138.

37 Cryns K, Van Camp G: Deafness genes and their diagnostic applications. Audiol Neurootol 2004;9:2–22.

38 Maeda Y, Fukushima K, Nishizaki K, Smith RJ: In vitro and in vivo suppression of *GJB2* expression by RNA interference. Hum Mol Genet 2005;14:1641–1650.

39 Yu Q, Wang Y, Chang Q, Wang J, Gong S, et al: Virally expressed connexin26 restores gap junction function in the cochlea of conditional *Gjb2* knockout mice. Gene Ther 2014;21:71–80.

40 Ruel J, Emery S, Nouvian R, Bersot T, Amilhon B, et al: Impairment of *SLC17A8* encoding vesicular glutamate transporter-3, VGLUT 3, underlies nonsyndromic deafness DFNA25 and inner hair cell dysfunction in null mice. Am J Hum Genet 2008;83:278–292.

41 Seal RP, Akil O, Yi E, Weber CM, Grant L, et al: Sensorineural deafness and seizures in mice lacking vesicular glutamate transporter 3. Neuron 2008;57:263–275.

42 Pan B, Géléoc GSG, Asai Y, Horwitz GC, Kurima K, et al: TMC1 and TMC2 are components of the mechanotransduction channel in hair cells of the mammalian inner ear. Neuron 2013;79:504–515.

43 Kawashima Y, Géléoc GSG, Kurima K, Labay V, Lelli A, et al: Mechanotransduction in mouse inner ear hair cells requires transmembrane channel-like genes. J Clin Invest 2011;121:4796–4809.

44 Zhao Y, Wang D, Zong L, Zhao F, Guan L, et al: A novel DFNA36 mutation in *TMC1* orthologous to the Beethoven *(Bth)* mouse associated with autosomal dominant hearing loss in a Chinese family. PLoS One 2014;9:e97064.

45 Lentz JJ, Jodelka FM, Hinrich AJ, McCaffrey KE, Farris HE, et al: Rescue of hearing and vestibular function by antisense oligonucleotides in a mouse model of human deafness. Nat Med 2013;19:345–350.

46 Izumikawa M, Minoda R, Kawamoto K, Abrashkin KA, Swiderski DL, et al: Auditory hair cell replacement and hearing improvement by *Atoh1* gene therapy in deaf mammals. Nat Med 2005;11:271–276.

47 Praetorius M, Hsu C, Baker K, Brough DE, Plinkert P, Staecker H: Adenovector-mediated hair cell regeneration is affected by promoter type. Acta Otolaryngol 2010;130:215–222.

48 Kesser BW, Hashisaki GT, Holt JR: Gene transfer in human vestibular epithelia and the prospects for inner ear gene therapy. Laryngoscope 2008;118:821–831.

49 Kesser BW, Hashisaki GT, Fletcher K, Eppard H, Holt JR: An in vitro model system to study gene therapy in the human ear. Gene Ther 2007;14:1121–1131.

50 Hakuba N, Watabe K, Hyodo J, Ohashi T, Eto Y, et al: Adenovirus-mediated overexpression of a gene prevents hearing loss and progressive inner hair cell loss after transient cochlear ischemia in gerbils. Gene Ther 2003;10:426–433.

51 Havenith S, Versnel H, Agterberg MJ, de Groot JC, Sedee RJ, et al: Spiral ganglion cell survival after round window membrane application of brain-derived neurotrophic factor using gelfoam as carrier. Hear Res 2011;272:168–177.

52 Leake PA, Stakhovskaya O, Hetherington A, Rebscher SJ, Bonham B: Effects of brain-derived neurotrophic factor (BDNF) and electrical stimulation on survival and function of cochlear spiral ganglion neurons in deafened, developing cats. J Assoc Res Otolaryngol 2013; 14:187–211.

53 Wan G, Gómez-Casati ME, Gigliello AR, Liberman MC, Corfas G: Neurotrophin-3 regulates ribbon synapse density in the cochlea and induces synapse regeneration after acoustic trauma. Elife 2014; 3:e03564.

54 Wise AK, Tu T, Atkinson PJ, Flynn BO, Sgro BE, et al: The effect of deafness duration on neurotrophin gene therapy for spiral ganglion neuron protection. Hear Res 2011;278:69–76.

55 Shibata SB, Di Pasquale G, Cortez SR, Chiorini JA, Raphael Y: Gene transfer using bovine adeno-associated virus in the guinea pig cochlea. Gene Ther 2009; 16:990–997.

56 Wu J, Liu B, Fan J, Zhu Q, Wu J: Study of protective effect on rat cochlear spiral ganglion after blast exposure by adenovirus-mediated human β-nerve growth factor gene. Am J Otolaryngol 2011;32: 8–12.

Omar Akil, PhD
Department of Otolaryngology – Head and Neck Surgery
University of California San Francisco
533 Parnassus Avenue, Room U490A
San Francisco, CA 94143-0526 (USA)
E-Mail oakil@ohns.ucsf.edu

Author Index

Subject Index